Research in Criminology

Series Editors
Alfred Blumstein
David P. Farrington

Research in Criminology

Understanding and Controlling Crime: Toward A New Research Strategy
D.P. Farrington, L.E. Ohlin and J.Q. Wilson

The Social Ecology of Crime
J.M. Byrne and R.J. Sampson (Eds.)

The Reasoning Criminal: Rational Choice Perspectives on Offending
D.B. Cornish and R.V. Clarke (Eds.)

The Social Contexts of Criminal Sentencing
Martha A. Myers and Susette M. Talarico

Predicting Recidivism Using Survival Models
Peter Schmidt and Ann Dryden Witte

Coping, Behavior, and Adaptation in Prison Inmates
Edward Zamble and Frank Porporino

Prison Crowding: A Psychological Perspective
Paul B. Paulus

Peter Schmidt
Ann Dryden Witte

Predicting Recidivism Using Survival Models

Springer-Verlag
New York Berlin Heidelberg
London Paris Tokyo

Peter Schmidt
Department of Economics, Michigan State University, East Lansing, Michigan 48824, USA.

Ann Dryden Witte
Department of Economics, Wellesley College, Wellesley, Massachusetts 02181, USA.
Research Associate, National Bureau of Economic Research, Cambridge, Massachusetts 02138, USA.

Series Editors
Alfred Blumstein
School of Urban and Public Affairs, Carnegie-Mellon University, Pittsburgh, Pennsylvania 15213, USA.

David P. Farrington
Institute of Criminology, University of Cambridge, Cambridge CB3 9DT, England.

Library of Congress Cataloging-in-Publication Data
Schmidt, Peter, 1947–
Predicting recidivism using survival models.
(Research in criminology)
1. Recidivism—Statistical methods.
2. Criminal behavior, Prediction of. I. Witte, Ann D.
II. Title. III. Series.
HV6049.S295 1988 364.3 87-20551

Softcover reprint of the hardcover 1st edition 1988

Typeset by Best-set Typesetter Ltd., Hong Kong.

9 8 7 6 5 4 3 2 1

ISBN-13:978-1-4612-8343-0 e-ISBN-13:978-1-4612-3772-3
DOI:10.1007/978-1-4612-3772-3

Preface

Our interest in the statistical modeling of data on the timing of recidivism began in the mid 1970s when we were both junior members of the economics department at the University of North Carolina. At that time, methods of analyzing qualitative and limited variables were being developed rapidly in the econometric literature, and we became interested in finding a suitable application for these new methods. Data on the timing of recidivism offered unique and interesting statistical challenges, such as skewness of the distribution and the presence of censoring. Being young and foolish, we decided it would be fun to try something "really" difficult. And, being young and ignorant, we were blissfully unaware of the concurrent developments in the statistical modeling of survival times that were then appearing in the biostatistics, operations research, and criminological literatures.

In the course of some earlier research, we had learned that the North Carolina Department of Correction had an unusually well-developed data base on their inmates. We approached the Department and asked if they would be interested in working with us to develop models that would predict when their former charges would return to their custody. They agreed because they were interested in using such models to evaluate rehabilitative programs and alternative prison management systems and to help project future prison populations.

We delivered our first set of models to the Department in 1976 and provided updated versions of some of the models in 1978. The Department used our models for a variety of internal purposes in the late 1970s and early 1980s. In 1982, with the publication of Greenwood's monograph heralding the advantages of selective incapacitation, the North Carolina legislature and other policy makers became interested in our models and their possible usefulness in implementing a policy of selective incapacitation.

By the mid 1980s, the models had outlived their usefulness; they no longer predicted satisfactorily for random samples of releasees. The Department asked if we would be interested in developing new models for them. We agreed for two reasons. First, there had been a number of new developments in the modeling of survival times in the statistical, operations research, and criminological literatures, and we wanted to explore the usefulness of these developments for modeling recidivism. Conversely, we felt that some aspects of our earlier work (especially the use of individual characteristics as explanatory variables) had been insufficiently appreciated in the criminological literature, and we wanted to incorporate them into the more recently developed models in criminology. Second, we wanted to evaluate the accuracy of individual predictions of recidivism. We were (and still are) skeptical that one can predict recidivism accurately enough, at the individual level, to justify a program of selective incapacitation, but we wanted to try to do so using the most promising models we could devise.

Somewhat to our surprise, the developments in survival modeling that turned out to be most useful to us were found in the criminological literature, and not in the literatures of statistics, operations research, or econometrics. Statistical modeling in criminology has by now attained sufficient sophistication that it contains unique and important insights; some of these are likely to be useful in other fields of application as well as in criminology. Indeed, one of the important findings of our research is that "off the shelf" techniques from the biostatistical and operations research literatures do not necessarily work very well with criminological data.

The most successful models presented in this book combine two distinct strands of the criminological literature on survival times. Unsurprisingly, the first such strand is our own previous work. Perhaps reflecting our background as economists (who are very fond of multiple regressions, or anything that resembles a multiple regression), we have always included explanatory variables in our models. We have found it surprising that most other researchers who have used survival models in criminology have not included explanatory variables in their models. The reason for this is not entirely clear, though it may just reflect the scarcity of release cohort data with any reliable information on the characteristics of the releasees or other variables that could explain recidivism. We believe strongly in the value of explanatory variables in survival models in criminology. The use of explanatory variables allows one to make statements about the way in which survival time is influenced by individual characteristics, criminal history, or structural variables, and it also allows one to make predictions for individuals and not just for random samples of releasees.

A second aspect of our previous work that is reflected in this book is the selection of a distribution for survival time. Most data on time until recidivism have a nonmonotonic hazard rate, and it is therefore important to pick a distribution that allows this possibility. Most survival models from biostatistics or operations research, and many of the models previously used in criminology, assume distributions that allow only a monotonic hazard rate. Our previous research used the lognormal distribution, for which the hazard rate first rises and then falls, matching the pattern found in the data. We find this to be a useful distribution again in the more sophisticated models developed in this book.

The other strand of the criminological literature that strongly influenced our current work is well represented by the publications of Maltz and his colleagues. Since the mid 1970s, these researchers have estimated "split population models" that explicitly account for the fact that not every individual will eventually fail; the probability of eventual failure is a parameter to be estimated along with the distribution of failure times for those individuals who will eventually fail. Split models have not been used much outside of criminology, though it seems to us that they could be. For example, models seeking to predict loan default should arguably be split models, as most loans do not eventually end in default.

The most innovative feature of our present work is the specification of split population models with explanatory variables. We parameterize both the probability of eventual failure and the distribution of time until failure for those who will ultimately fail. This allows us to make separate statements about the effects of individual characteristics on these two different aspects of return to prison. For example, we find that race and sex affect the probability of eventual recidivism but not its timing, whereas two indicators of the nature of the previous offense affect the timing of recidivism (for the eventual recidivists) but not the probability of eventual recidivism. Distinctions of this type are important in a variety of contexts. For example, in the career criminal paradigm, one may wish to distinguish the determinants of participation and frequency. As another example, in the loan default problem one might wish to distinguish the determinants of the probability of default from the determinants of the timing of default.

We hope and expect that the next few years will see a growing interest in (and application of) survival models that include individual characteristics as explanatory variables. Furthermore, we hope that split models and models with nonmonotonic hazard rates will find uses both in criminology and in other social science research. This seems to us to be a very promising path of research, and this book is intended as a step along that path.

In order to facilitate further work on the application of survival models to data on recidivism, we have made our data available through the Inter-university Consortium for Political and Social Research (ICPSR) at the University of Michigan. The data are also available on floppy diskette from the first author; this offer expires 5 years after the publication of this book.

The work reported here would not have been possible without the generous support of the National Institute of Justice (NIJ) and the North Carolina Department of Correction (NCDOC). In particular, we would like to thank Richard Laymon and Dick Linster of NIJ and Ken Parker of NCDOC.

We gratefully acknowledge the helpful comments of Richard Berk, Al Blumstein, Kurt Brannas, Jan Chaiken, David Farrington, Brian Forst,

Dennis Hoffman, Dick Linster, Michael Maltz, John Monohan, John Rolph, and William Spelman on this manuscript or parts thereof. We would like to thank Kari Peterson and Lisa Schineller for research assistance and Helen Blatt for typing. Finally, we thank our families for their patience with the disruptions that the preparation of a book entails.

Contents

Prediction in criminology has always been an important topic, and it will continue to be important in the foreseeable future.

FARRINGTON and TARLING (1985, p. 268)

Future development of prediction models should be aimed at improving the classification of offenders in terms of their frequency of offending and their residual career length. While these career developments are not directly observable, their values can be inferred using statistical techniques that analyze time to recidivism.

BLUMSTEIN et al. (1986, vol. 1, p. 9)

One of the most important uses of recidivism analyses is in estimating the characteristics of offender populations. Knowing how many people recidivate, the frequency with which they do so, when they terminate their criminal careers, and other characteristics of their offending behavior is useful in many policy-related areas.

MALTZ (1984, p. 26)

1
Introduction

Overview

During the 1970s and early 1980s, evidence accumulated indicating that a relatively small group of offenders committed most serious offenses. These findings, coupled with increasing pressures on the budgets of criminal justice agencies, led to calls for more effective use of the public expenditures for crime control by identifying and incarcerating the most serious and persistent offenders.[1] These calls for selective incapacitation have focused attention on the causes of crime and on the problem of predicting which individuals will commit crimes in the future.

The research community has responded by producing a large number of articles and books on the prediction of crime, the causes of crime, and criminal careers. Several books have been written that summarize what we know about the causes of crime[2] and how well we are able to predict criminality,[3] while most articles tend to report the results of particular studies. In this book, we take a middle ground between broadly synthetic works and much more narrowly focused articles. Our focus is primarily on statistical methodology. More specifically, we assess various parametric and nonparametric methods for predicting whether and when a released prisoner will return to crime. The relevant statistical methodology was developed mainly in the operations research and biostatistical literatures, and the appropriate statistical models are generally referred to as "survival time" or "failure time" models. Throughout this book, we will use these two terms interchangeably to refer to statistical models designed to analyze the timing of events of interest.

In the last 10 years or so, there has been increasing interest in using these

---

[1] For example, see the extremely influential work of Greenwood (1982).

[2] For example, see Schmidt and Witte (1984, Part II), Wilson and Herrnstein (1985), and Blumstein et al. (1986).

[3] For example, see Maltz (1984), Schmidt and Witte (1984, Part I), Farrington and Tarling (1985), and Gottfredson and Tonry (1987).

methods to analyze the criminal careers or recidivism of previous offenders.[4] However, as noted by the National Academy of Sciences' Panel on Research on Criminal Careers, "failure-rate models have been applied only rarely to criminal justice prediction problems ... and so the extra statistical power they can provide in separately predicting frequency rates for active offenders and dropout rates are not yet widely understood and appreciated" (Blumstein, Cohen, Roth, and Visher, 1986, p. 171). We hope that this book will help to broaden the appeal of survival models and that it will lead to their wider use in civil and criminal justice research. We believe that survival analysis will be one of the major methodological innovations in justice research during the next decade, in the same way as models for the analysis of qualitative dependent variables (such as log linear, logit, and probit models) were during the last decade.

Various parametric and nonparametric survival models have previously been used in criminal justice applications. However, the choice of technique often appears to be a matter of convenience rather than the result of careful thought and analysis. Some researchers have incorporated individual characteristics into their models, while others have not. We believe that it is now time to consider carefully which survival models are most appropriate for criminal justice applications and develop guidelines that will allow the applied researcher to choose an appropriate technique for his or her particular application. In this book, we carry out extensive tests to determine which survival model best accounts for the length of time until a released prisoner returns to crime. We see this work as serving two main purposes. First, and perhaps most importantly, it illustrates the important issues that the applied researcher should consider when choosing a survival model. Second, it makes a substantive contribution to the literature on the prediction of recidivism; it shows how to make such predictions and provides evidence on how well we can expect to predict recidivism.

The analysis of recidivism has represented the most frequent use of survival models in criminal justice research, and it seems likely that this will continue to be the case. Focusing on this application of these techniques should, therefore, be particularly useful. However, survival models have potentially much broader applications in civil and criminal justice. For example, they could be used to analyze when individuals file their tax returns, the length of time needed to "clear" police cases, or the length of time needed to process court cases.

As noted earlier, survival models are designed to analyze the length of

---

[4] As far as we are aware, the earliest use of survival models in criminal justice was by Carr-Hill and Carr-Hill (1972). There was a rather substantial amount of work with various parametric techniques in the late 1970s. More recently, a number of researchers have used the proportional hazards model developed by Cox (1972). See Maltz (1984), Schmidt and Witte (1984), or the section Previous Use of Survival Analysis in Justice Research for reviews of this literature.

time until an event occurs. In the operations research literature, such techniques have been used extensively to study the reliability (time until failure) of electronic components. In the biostatistical literature, the length of time that a patient survives after treatment is of primary interest. Our own work using these methods to analyze recidivism dates back to the mid 1970s, and it convinces us that the proper and productive use of these techniques in justice research requires the careful and rather sophisticated analysis of large and detailed sets of data. In this book, we carry out such analyses. We seek to explain and predict the length of time that elapses between an individual's release from incarceration and his or her return to prison, using data on two cohorts of releasees from North Carolina's state prisons.

The ability to predict recidivism can aid criminal justice decision-making and planning. For example, a judge often uses information on the likelihood of future return to crime in deciding the sentence to impose. Parole boards may also use such predictions when deciding whether or not to grant early release. Similarly, predictions of recidivism can improve criminal justice planning. For example, correctional planners are better able to project future needs when they are better informed about the likely return of "old friends" whom they have incarcerated in the past.

While our study is somewhat narrowly focused on the future criminal activities of prison releasees, we believe that some of the models we develop have far broader applications. For example, one of the models that we present in Chapter 7 allows one to separate the effects of explanatory variables on the probability of ever committing an offense from their effects on the frequency of offending for those who do become involved in crime. As noted in the recent report of the National Academy of Sciences' Panel on Research on Criminal Careers (Blumstein et al., 1986), the factors affecting participation in crime and those affecting the frequency of offenses for those who do participate may be quite different. For example, being black appears to increase the probability of offending, but does not appear to influence the frequency of offending. To date, such inferences have been drawn using relatively unsophisticated techniques. We hope that our work will help to advance the state of the statistical art for this type of research.

In this chapter, we provide a brief overview of the important issues in prediction and career criminal research, and we discuss previous work that has used survival analysis to study criminal justice topics. The outline of the chapter is as follows. In the section Prediction in Criminology, we consider the use of prediction in criminal justice research, and we discuss some of the important issues currently being debated in the criminological literature on prediction. In the section The Career Criminal Paradigm, we consider the "career criminal" paradigm and its relationship to our work. In the section Previous Use of Survival Analysis in Justice Research, we review previous research that has used survival models to analyze the timing of events that are of interest to criminologists. The final section of this chapter provides a synopsis of the book. It is our preview of coming attractions.

Prediction in Criminology

Criminologists have a long history of interest in prediction, presumably because the ability to predict outcomes accurately would be of immense practical use. The administration of the criminal justice system involves a large number of decisions, many of which might be improved if decision-makers were better informed about what the future is likely to hold. For example, police officers must decide whether or not to arrest a suspicious character, prosecutors must decide whether or not to bring a case to trial, and judges must decide whether or not to grant pre-trial release and what type of sentence to impose on convicted offenders. Correctional officials must decide on the security level and the activities of their charges, and parole boards must decide whether to release an inmate before the expiration of his or her sentence. Most criminal justice decision-makers base their decisions at least in part on their prediction of the likely future actions of the individual whose fate they are considering.

It is surely true that most predictions of the likely future actions of suspected offenders are made informally on the basis of experience or clinical judgment. However, there has recently been increased interest in statistical or actuarial predictions. This is partly because statistical predictions may be justified on objective scientific grounds, and partly because of an accumulation of evidence that statistical predictions tend to be more accurate than clinical and other informal methods and can provide a valuable decision aid to criminal justice decision-makers.[5]

There have been several recent reviews of the prediction literature. We will summarize the conclusions of these reviews, adding a few insights of our own.[6] In the sections that follow, we will first discuss some of the ethical issues involved in making and using predictions in the administration of the criminal justice system. We will then turn to the more technical issues of sample selection, variable selection, and selection of a statistical methodology. We will end the section with a discussion of reasonable goals for prediction in criminology.

---

[5] For example, see Monahan (1981) and Gottfredson and Gottfredson (1986). Gottfredson and Gottfredson (1986, p. 247) conclude that "in virtually every decision-making situation for which the issue has been studied, it has been found that statistically developed predictive devices outperform human judgments."

[6] The reviews we will draw on most heavily are Farrington (1987), Farrington and Tarling (1985), Gottfredson (1987), and Gottfredson and Gottfredson (1986).

ETHICAL ISSUES

The possibility of using formal methods of prediction in criminal justice decision-making raises the question of when and in what ways it is ethical to do so. This question has been much discussed in the criminological literature. Good summaries include Blumstein et al. (1986), Farrington (1987), Morris and Miller (1985) and Tonry (1987). We will provide only a brief summary of some of the views expressed and a few opinions of our own.

The most obvious set of ethical concerns has to do with which possible uses of prediction should be allowable. For example, proponents of selective incapacitation, such as Greenwood (1982), clearly find it acceptable to treat certain individuals more harshly than they would otherwise be treated on the basis of a prediction of their likely future behavior. Not everyone agrees with this position. Morris and Miller (1985) believe that an increase in penalties because of a prediction of likely future criminality is acceptable only if the punishment is not increased beyond that which would be justified as "deserved" independently of such a prediction. Others, such as Gottfredson and Gottfredson (1986), would support the use of prediction to select individuals for less severe punishment ("selective deinstitutionalization"), but they would not support any use of prediction to select individuals for more severe punishment. Wilkins (1985) is comfortable in making predictions that will be used to determine the punishment for convicted offenders, but he is not willing to make predictions about who is likely to become an offender.

In this work, we take no specific position on this debate. (Indeed, in writing this section, it quickly became apparent that our views differed.) In our previous work, we never made predictions for individuals, even though we made group predictions that were derived from such individual predictions.[7] So far as we know, the North Carolina Department of Correction (for whom we carried out this earlier work) has also refrained from using our models to predict whether a given individual would return to crime. In this book, we again construct models that could be used to make predictions for individuals, and we make such predictions explicitly in Chapter 8. However, our interest in doing so is purely scientific: we wish to investigate how well it is possible to predict at the individual level. Though we are able to predict reasonably well by the current standards of prediction in criminology, it should be recognized that the ability of previous researchers to predict criminal justice outcomes has not been great. Our levels of false positive and false negative results are high enough that it would be very hard to justify differential treatment of individuals on the basis of our predictions, at least for more than a very small percentage of the sample. We do not dismiss the importance of a discussion of the

---

[7] See Schmidt and Witte (1976, 1978, 1984).

ethics of a policy of selective incapacitation or of other similar policies, but we believe that the point is basically moot until models are developed that predict more accurately than is currently possible.

Assuming that the acceptable uses of prediction in criminal justice were decided, we would still be left with the issue of deciding what information should be used in making these predictions. In the usual settings in criminal justice, the available information generally consists of extensive data on the attributes, experiences, and activities of the individuals. The use of such information for prediction generally involves two steps. First, a set of individual data is used to estimate a model. Second, the model is used, together with information on an individual, to predict the individual's future behavior. In our opinion, ethical questions about the type of information that should be used arise only in the second step of this process. However, it is important to emphasize that the only way to be sure that an unacceptable piece of information (e.g., race) is *not included* in the second step of this process is to *include* it in the first step. This is a point that seems to be missed often, so it is perhaps worthy of explanation.

In step one of the prediction process, when estimating the prediction model, we believe that all information relevant to the behavioral outcome of interest should be used. This is basically just a matter of good statistical practice, since the omission of relevant variables from the model will lead to biased parameter estimates if the omitted variables are correlated with the included variables. For example, if race is omitted from the model, and if it is correlated with education, the estimated coefficient of education will reflect both its "true" coefficient (holding race constant) and also a bias term; the bias term arises from the effect of race being implicitly assigned to those included variables (such as education) that are correlated with race. The use of such biased coefficients can be argued to be discriminatory, just as the use of race to make predictions would be, because it amounts to choosing the variables used in prediction at least in part on the basis of their correlation with race. For example, the omission of race from the model will bias the coefficient of education if blacks return to prison sooner than whites and if blacks are on average less well educated. Thus, education will be a spuriously good predictor of parole success. If so, a parole board using these results will tend to release prisoners with high levels of education, and these prisoners will be predominantly white. The only way to avoid such an outcome is to include race as an explanatory variable in the first (estimation of the model) stage of the prediction process. We therefore support the use of such controversial variables as race, ethnic group, sex, age, or religion when estimating a prediction model, if these variables help to explain the behavior that we are seeking to predict. For example, in our work, we seek to predict the return to prison of releasees from North Carolina's state prisons. Race and sex are strongly related to return to prison. Because this is so, we use such variables when estimating our models.

The second step in prediction is to use the model estimated in step one to predict future behavior. At this stage, ethical questions certainly arise about what kinds of information should be used. Consider the admonition of the Panel on Research on Criminal Careers (Blumstein et al. 1986, p. 8): "Characteristics such as race, ethnicity, and religion are especially unacceptable as candidate predictors because they have no relationship to blameworthiness, ... and their use affronts basic social values." We quite agree, and we would strongly oppose using information on race or sex in making predictions from our models for criminal justice decision-making. The essential point is that not every variable used in estimating the model needs to be used when making predictions from the model; one can simply ignore the information on unacceptable variables and use the model and the information on acceptable variables to make predictions. The important statistical and practical issue is how much the failure to use unacceptable information in step two compromises our ability to make accurate predictions. We explore this issue in Chapter 8. To do so, we first predict recidivism using our fully specified model and information on all variables in the model, including race and sex. We then make predictions using the parameter estimates from our fully specified model, but ignoring the information on race and sex. Encouragingly, we find that there is little loss of predictive power as a result of choosing not to use the available information on these two variables.[8]

What Sample Should Be Used to Estimate the Model?

Prediction models should be estimated using data on a sample of a large number of individuals, and the group of individuals who make up the sample should be as representative as possible of the group for whom predictions are to be made. For example, when the North Carolina Department of Correction asked us to estimate a model that would allow them to predict return to their system, we asked them to supply us with entire release cohorts. For our present work, we used data on two such release cohorts: (1) all individuals released from prison in North Carolina between July 1, 1977 and June 30, 1978, and (2) all individuals released between July 1, 1979 and June 30, 1980. Each of these cohorts contains approximately 9,500 individuals; they certainly qualify as large.

It is generally harder to decide whether a data set is representative of the group for which predictions are to be made. In part, this is simply because one may not know exactly for which groups predictions will be made, and it is hard to find a representative sample without knowing what it is supposed

[8] See Petersilia and Turner (1987) for an extended discussion of the effect of omitting variables that are correlated with race when making predictions of recidivism.

to represent. For example, at this point we do not know how (or even whether) the North Carolina Department of Correction will use the models developed in this book. The Department used the models that we provided in 1976 and 1978 in diverse ways, such as evaluation of rehabilitative programs and projection of future prison populations. Not all such possible uses could be anticipated at the time the data were collected. Under these circumstances, the best way in which to proceed was to use a random sample of releasees (e.g., a release cohort). At least it is clear what group this represents. Furthermore, when it is time to make predictions, it may be possible to consider the ways in which the group for which predictions are made differs from a release cohort.

A related point is that the careful incorporation of individual characteristics as explanatory variables may help the model to predict accurately for groups that differ systematically from the sample used in estimation. At least the model can then correct for the differences between the two groups in the values of these individual characteristics, and this is almost certain to result in improved predictions. The extent to which we find this to be true in our analyses will be discussed in detail in Chapter 8.

Selection of a Criterion Variable

To estimate a prediction model, it is obviously necessary to decide exactly what variable one will seek to predict. The criterion variable which we analyzed is the length of time between release from North Carolina's state prisons and return thereto. This dependent variable is clearly preferable to the much more commonly used binary criterion variable, which simply indicates whether or not an individual returns to prison during the follow-up period.[9] Blumstein et al. (1986), Farrington and Tarling (1985), Stollmack and Harris (1974), Sechrest, White, and Brown (1979), Harris, Kaylan, and Maltz (1981), Maltz (1984), and Schmidt and Witte (1984) all argue that a dependent variable that contains information on the timing of recidivism is preferable to a simple binary (yes/no) indicator of recidivism. Basically, there are two such arguments. First, from a statistical point of view, the timing of recidivism contains valuable information, and it is statistically inefficient to ignore such information. Second, estimating the distribution of the length of time until recidivism allows one to predict the rate of recidivism for any desired period after release, not just for the particular follow-up period found in the data used to estimate the model.

Our choice to analyze the timing of *return to prison* is open to criticism and certainly restricts the way in which our results should be used. If our

---

[9] For recent examples of the use of such a binary criterion variable, see Berk and Rauma (1983), Farrington and Morris (1983), Farrington (1985), Black and Spinks (1985), Ghali (1982), and Menard and Covey (1983).

goal were simply to provide a planning and evaluation tool for the North Carolina Department of Correction, this criterion variable is clearly of interest. However, if our concerns are broader (for example, understanding the factors leading to a resumption of criminal activity), then this criterion variable is open to serious challenge. The results we obtain using this criterion variable will reflect not only the behavior of the individual, but also the decisions of the criminal justice system that lead to his or her reincarceration.[10] The same problem would arise if our criterion variable were time until rearrest or time until reconviction, of course, but presumably in a less serious form as there are less criminal justice system decisions prior to rearrest or reconviction than there are prior to return to prison.

Because we would certainly prefer to analyze the timing of return to criminal activity if that were observable, another possibility is to use self-report information to define the criterion variable.[11] However, self-report information suffers from its own inaccuracies. For example, Weis (1986) reports that blacks underreport their criminal activity in self-reports much more than whites do. If this is so, the estimated effect of race will reflect both its "true" effect on the criminal decision and the difference in the extent to which blacks and whites choose to report these decisions (i.e., response bias). This is not different in principle from the fact that, in our models, the estimated effect of race reflects both its "true" effect on the criminal decision and the effect of the individual's race on his or her treatment by the criminal justice system.

We analyzed the timing of return to prison in North Carolina because this was the only definition of recidivism that our data would support. In interpreting our results, we will be careful to recognize that the estimates we obtain reflect the decisions of releasees, victims, police, prosecutors, and judges. The information the estimates contain is clearly of interest, but it is impossible to separate out the effects of the various decision-makers.

Use and Selection of Explanatory Variables

We estimate three types of models. In Chapter 4, we estimate models that use no individual characteristics. Such models have been very popular in criminal justice applications, particularly in studies of recidivism.[12] These models contain no explanatory variables; they are simply models of the marginal distribution of time until recidivism.

---

[10] See Carr-Hill and Stern (1979), Witte (1980), Schmidt and Witte (1984), and Blumstein et al. (1986) for discussions of the interpretation of the parameter estimates in models of various criminal justice outcomes.

[11] See Weis (1986) for an excellent discussion of self-reports and other measures of criminal activity.

[12] See Maltz (1984) for a thorough survey of this literature.

In Chapter 5, we estimate models that contain no individual characteristics as explanatory variables, but which do allow for individual differences in a very simple way. Specifically, these "split models" postulate that there are two types of individuals: those who would eventually return to prison and those who would never return to prison.[13] In these models, the probability of eventual failure becomes an additional parameter to be estimated.

Finally, in Chapters 6 and 7, we estimate models that incorporate individual characteristics as explanatory variables. Our selection of explanatory variables is based on data availability and the results of previous studies of recidivism. For the purpose of providing the North Carolina Department of Correction with a useful decision-making tool, this method of selection does not appear unreasonable. On the other hand, if our primary purpose was to determine the causes of crime, it presumably would be preferable to choose explanatory variables on the basis of some theory, as Farrington and Tarling (1985) have pointed out. A difficulty with this suggestion, however, is that there is no comprehensive theory of crime that finds general agreement among criminologists.[14]

We believe that one of the major contributions of our work is the development and use of survival time models that explicitly incorporate explanatory variables. The biostatistics literature has used such "covariates" for some time, and it is surprising to us that the criminal justice literature that uses survival methods ignores explanatory variables by and large. While we have used survival models with explanatory variables since the mid 1970s, this was clearly the exception rather than the rule.[15] Even in the 1980s, there has been remarkably little use of covariates in survival models; they seem to have been used only in the context of Cox's "proportional hazards model."[16]

It is important to note that there are two rather different senses in which

---

[13] Again, Maltz (1984) provides a good survey.

[14] As an example of disagreement about theories of crime causation, consider the controversy over the so-called economic theory of crime, for which Schmidt and Witte (1984) provide a useful survey.

[15] For examples of our work, see Schmidt and Witte (1976, 1978, 1979) and Witte and Schmidt (1977). For examples of survival analyses of recidivism that do not use individual characteristics, see Carr-Hill and Carr-Hill (1972), Stollmack and Harris (1974), Maltz and McCleary (1977), Harris and Moitra (1978), and Bloom (1979).

[16] Schmidt and Witte (1984) contains our more recent work. Witte et al. (1982), Sherman and Berk (1984), and Rhodes and Matsuba (1985) provide examples of the use of the proportional hazards model. Work on models without covariates has also continued, and Maltz (1984) provides a good summary of this work. Chaiken and Rolph (1981) provide some additional work which does not explicitly incorporate explanatory variables. Their paper also provides an interesting discussion of the difficulties they encountered when attempting to incorporate explanatory variables.

the use of explanatory variables may improve predictions of recidivism. First, by reducing the variance of the prediction for each individual in a group, we should reduce the variance of the prediction for the group average (recidivism rate). An analysis of survival time without using explanatory variables amounts to an analysis of its *marginal* distribution, whereas an analysis using explanatory variables amounts to an analysis of the distribution of survival time *conditional* on these variables. It is a standard result that the variance of the conditional distribution is less than the variance of the marginal distribution. In a linear regression model, the ratio of these two variances is one minus the R^2 of the regression (the proportion of the variance of the dependent variable not "explained" by the explanatory variables). Similar considerations apply in more complicated models, such as the ones we use here; the variance of our predictions of the survival time will be reduced to the extent that we can explain the variance of survival time with observable explanatory variables.

The second sense in which the use of explanatory variables may improve predictions of recidivism is that it allows one to correct for differences between the group used to estimate the model and the group for which predictions are to be made. As a simple example, suppose one has estimated a model using data on a random sample of releasees (of all ages), but wishes to make predictions of the rate of recidivism for a group of youthful offenders. There is little hope of accurate predictions unless the statistical model contained age as an explanatory variable. In a more detailed example, we will later (in Chapter 8) report results of analyses of time until recidivism for random samples of individuals released from prison in North Carolina in 1978 and 1980. The rate of recidivism is higher for 1980 releasees than for 1978 releasees. When we fit models without explanatory variables to the 1978 data, the models consistently underpredict the rate of recidivism in the 1980 data. On the other hand, when we fit models which use individual characteristics as explanatory variables to the 1978 data, the models predict the 1980 releasees' recidivism quite accurately. In other words, differences in *observed* characteristics of the releasees appear to explain adequately the differences in recidivism rates of the 1978 and 1980 cohorts.

There are two other obvious reasons why it may be worthwhile to include individual characteristics in models of time until recidivism. First, it enables one to make statements about the effects of demographic or environmental variables on return to prison, and these may be interesting. For example, we will later report results indicating that the time until recidivism is signficantly related to age, race, sex, marital status, alcohol or drug abuse, the number of previous convictions, the length of previous sentence, and the nature of previous offense. As noted earlier, these results must be interpreted with care as they are the outcome of numerous decisions by diverse decison-makers. However, they may still be informative for both research and policy. Second, the use of individual characteristics allows one to make predictions of the probability of recidivism for *individuals* as well as for groups. Such predictions are of interest as proposals for selective incapacitation have come to be discussed quite seriously (for example, see Greenwood, 1982), and as attempts have been made to systematize bail, prosecution, sentencing, and parole decisions (see Gottfredson & Gottfredson, 1986). We can also make statements about *how well* we can predict recidivism at the individual level. For example, in our data, the fit of the models is sufficiently loose (i.e., the percentage of the variability in timing of recidivism explained by the models is sufficiently low) that we would not seriously contemplate using them to implement a policy of selective incapacitation.

Selection of a Statistical Model

In the present context, the selection of a statistical model amounts to the specification of the distribution of the criterion variable, conditional on the individual characteristics used as explanatory variables. Recall that we have selected the length of time until a releasee returns to prison as our criterion variable. The distribution of this variable contains a number of unusual features that call for care in its statistical analysis. For one thing, the distribution is skewed to the right, with most individuals returning to prison doing so during the first two years after release. Return during the first few months is not common because criminal justice processing generally causes a lag between the time that an individual returns to crime and the time that he or she shows up in criminal justice records, as pointed out by Carr-Hill and Carr-Hill (1972).[17] This lag would be far shorter if arrest, rather than return to prison, were used as the criterion variable.

A second notable feature of time until recidivism is that its distribution is censored on the right. Although our follow-up periods are quite long, ranging from 46 to 81 months, we do not observe return to prison for all individuals during the follow-up period. It is inappropriate either to drop the individuals who do not return to prison or to set their date of return at the end of the follow-up period.[18] The proper treatment of the censoring problem is a standard topic in the statistical survival time literature; the

[17] It is interesting that Carr-Hill and Carr-Hill (1972) chose to simply subtract one month from the reconviction date to reflect this lag. This is clearly not the appropriate way to handle this matter. It would be preferable to choose a distribution that allows the highest density to occur with a lag. Carr-Hill and Carr-Hill chose the exponential distribution, which does not allow this. In our work, we searched carefully for distributions which would reflect this feature of recidivism data.

[18] See Brannas and Eklof (1985) for a recent example of work that is statistically sophisticated but still ignores the censoring issue.

fact of censoring must be reflected in the likelihood function. We discuss this in detail in Chapter 3.

The final notable feature of survival times is that they are nonnegative by definition and may take on a wide range of values. Nonnegativity rules out many common distributions, such as the normal. However, a wide variety of potentially suitable distributions can be found in the survival model literature, and we consider a number of such distributions in Chapter 4.

What Are Realistic Goals for Prediction?

Although there is general acceptance of the proposition that statistical prediction is more accurate than informal or clinical prediction,[19] there is also pessimism concerning the ability of more sophisticated models to improve our abilty to predict recidivism. For example, both Gottfredson (1987) and Farrington and Tarling (1985) conclude that the use of more sophisticated statistical methods has not enabled criminal justice researchers to predict more accurately than Burgess (1928) did by giving equal weight to all explanatory variables. This is quite discouraging, and although Gottfredson, Farrington, and Tarling all call for further work on statistical methods, they were certainly not very optimistic regarding the ability of more sophisticated methods to achieve major improvements in prediction. Our own work is clearly centered on the use of more sophisticated methods, and thus we must come squarely to grips with the pessimism regarding our activity.

To assess the results of prediction research, one must first consider carefully what it might be possible to achieve in the best of all possible settings. Suppose that we had an extremely well developed theory of crime and were actually able to observe the actions of potential criminals. Further, suppose that we were able to collect information on all variables relevant to criminal activity. Assume that we had carefully chosen an appropriate statistical method and that we used this method and the data we had collected to estimate a model of criminality. How well should we expect this model to explain individual criminality?

We can only guess at the answer to this question, based on our experience with empirical work using individual data in other (perhaps related) fields. For example, there is a considerable body of work in the economics literature that seeks to explain an individual's wage rate on the basis of individual characteristics. The dependent variable is usually the logarithm of the wage rate; unlike many measures of recidivism, this is measured with relatively little error. The explanatory variables typically used are education, labor market experience, and a variety of characteris-

[19] See Monahan (1981), Farrington and Tarling (1985), and Gottfredson and Gottfredson (1986).

tics of the individual and (sometimes) of the job. These are also measured fairly accurately. Furthermore, it is safe to say that the relevant body of economic theory (the so-called "human capital" theory) is much more specific in its implications for the specification of wage equations than the relevant theory in criminology is in its implications for the specification of models of recidivism. Under these relatively favorable conditions, researchers are rarely able to explain over half of the variation in the dependent variable (log wage). Why? There are two basic reasons that are commonly cited. First, there is simply inherent randomness in individual decisions, and this element of uncertainty will remain even if we estimate the perfect model. Second, there are surely factors that affect individual decisions that we are unlikely to measure perfectly or even include in our model. For example, when estimating wage equations, we are unlikely to have perfect measures (or even any measures) of important variables such as ability or motivation. The more important such omitted variables are in explaining the criterion variable, the larger the random element that we observe will be.

We expect that criminal activity has a much larger random element than the wage rate and that we may *never* be able to explain more than 30% or so of the variation in typical variables representing criminality, even under ideal conditions. The reasons are straightforward. First, as just mentioned, it seems likely that the measurable outcomes of criminal decisions would be subject to far larger random or chance effects than wages. Second, we are likely to be forced to omit many more relevant explanatory variables when we estimate a crime equation than when we estimate a wage equation. Wages are determined by the joint decisions of employers and workers, whereas criminal activity requires the combination of proclivity and opportunity. Although it is quite possible to observe many relevant characteristics of employers and workers, it is much more difficult to measure the factors that lead to a willingness to commit criminal acts or to find variables that will accurately reflect the opportunities for crime that the potential criminal faces.

We are not discouraged by our likely inability to explain the majority of the variation in available measures of criminal activity. When the sample size is large, a model which explains only 10% of the variation in the dependent variable can yield statistically significant statements about the effects of explanatory variables. Such a model can also be useful from the point of view of both theory and policy. However, we believe that it is useful to consider the possible explanatory power of statistical models so that we evaluate prediction research against realistic rather than unattainable goals.

Prediction research in criminal justice has not taken place in the ideal setting described above. As might be expected, the level of explanatory power obtained has been far below 30%. After careful consideration of the literature, Gottfredson (1987, p.16) concludes that the proportion of the outcome variance explained rarely exceeds 15 to 20% and is most frequently lower. The studies that Gottfredson considered used overwhelmingly the traditional binary criterion variable. As discussed previously we use a more informative criterion variable, namely, the length of time from release to return to prison. With this dependent variable, we are seeking to explain not only who returns to crime, but also when they return. Since we are making greater demands on the model, we should expect to obtain lower explanatory power than if we were simply seeking to explain who returns to crime. As we report in Chapter 7, we obtain explanatory power which is quite similar (an equivalent of R^2 equal to .10 for 1978 and .12 for 1980) to that of most studies that use a binary criterion variable.[20] This is quite respectable in its own right. Furthermore, we conjecture (perhaps optimistically) that this level of explanatory power could be approximately doubled, with further experimentation with nonlinear effects of explanatory variables in our models. (We discuss the ways in which this might be done in Chapter 9.) Better data would allow further improvement.

The ultimate test of prediction research is not the proportion of the variance explained, but rather the ability to predict. After a very careful and useful survey of the literature, Farrington (1987, p. 54) concludes that "few well-designed prediction exercises will manage to keep both false positive and false negative rates below 50 percent." As we report in Chapter 8, we are able to do this. For example, in our 1978 validation sample, we have a false positive rate of 47% and a false negative rate of 28%. These results are encouraging because they indicate that we have succeeded in designing an effective prediction model by the usual standards of criminal justice research. However, the very high false positive rate clearly argues against using our predictions to impose more severe penalties on offenders.

The Career Criminal Paradigm

The publicity[21] surrounding the release of the report from the National Academy of Sciences' Panel on Research on Criminal Careers (Blumstein et al., 1986) has served to highlight the importance of research that carefully studies the offending patterns of individuals. The report develops

---

[20] Gottfredson and Gottfredson (1985) obtain values of R^2 ranging from .09 (using association analysis) to .14 (using multiple regression analysis). They used a binary criterion variable.

[21] When the panel report was released, there was a major conference of federal, state, and local officials and criminal justice researchers in Washington. Attorney General Edwin Meese III was the keynote speaker at the conference.

and uses the career criminal paradigm to study these patterns. This paradigm distinguishes four important aspects of the criminal choice:

1. *Participation*—the distinction between those who engage in crime and those who do not;
2. *Frequency*—the rate of criminal activity of those who are active;
3. *Seriousness* of offenses committed;
4. *Career length*—the length of time an offender is active. (Blumstein et al., 1986, p. 1)

As noted in the panel report, survival analysis is particularly appropriate for analyzing the frequency of offending and the length of criminal careers. These elements of criminal choice are relevant only for offenders. However, they are of central importance to criminal justice administrators and decision-makers since it is offenders with whom they must primarily deal. We hope that our work will help to answer the Academy's call for more research on survival techniques and will provide criminal justice practitioners with research that is useful.

The report does not call for the development of techniques that will allow one to look *simultaneously* at participation and the frequency of offending, but such techniques are clearly useful for research on criminal careers. At present, these two aspects of the criminal decision are generally studied separately with different statistical techniques. The models that we develop in Chapters 5 and 7 would allow one to estimate a single model that would address the participation and frequency aspects of criminal activity. The models developed in Chapter 7 allow different effects of explanatory variables on the probability of participation and the timing of criminal activity. This is important because existing research seems to indicate that different factors affect participation and frequency decisions.

Previous Use of Survival Analysis in Justice Research

The earliest use of survival analysis in justice research was apparently by Carr-Hill and Carr-Hill (1972). They estimated an exponential model (see the section The Exponential Distribution, Chapter 4) and a mixed exponential model that allows different processes to prevail for "quick reconvictors" and "slow reconvictors."[22] Their major interest was in the reconviction process rather than in recidivism, and they used no explanatory variables in their models.

Stollmack and Harris (1974) appear to be the first researchers who

---

[22] Greenberg (1978) suggests an extension of the Carr-Hill and Carr-Hill model to allow for three types of offenders: (1) those who take up a life of virtue; (2) those who are not committed to a life free of crime but who happen not to commit an offense; and (3) those who commit crimes and may or may not apprehended.

explicitly considered using survival analysis to model recidivism. Their specific interest was in the use of survival analysis to discern the effectiveness of various programs. Like Carr-Hill and Carr-Hill, they used an exponential model, and they did not consider explanatory variables.

Maltz and McCleary (1977) extended the work of Stollmack and Harris by considering a split population model. The population is (conceptually) divided into two groups, one which would eventually return to prison and one which would never do so. Maltz and McCleary follow Stollmack and Harris by assuming an exponential distribution for the eventual recidivists. They do not introduce explanatory variables into their model, but their adoption of a split population model implicitly assumes differences between individuals. This line of work has been continued by Maltz and his colleagues (Harris, Kaylan, & Maltz, 1981; Maltz, 1984; Maltz, 1978; Maltz, McCleary, & Pollock, 1979). This work has been very influential and has been commented on widely. For example, see the comments of Miley (1978), Lloyd and Joe (1979), and Stein and Lloyd (1981).

In Witte and Schmidt (1977), we considered several different models (based on different distributions) for time until recidivism, each of which explicitly contained explanatory variables. We developed these models in ignorance of earlier work in criminology, taking our inspiration instead from Amemiya and Boskin (1974). Amemiya and Boskin are economists who were interested in modeling the duration of welfare dependency. Like most economists, they were interested in the way in which personal characteristics affect behavior, and therefore they explicitly introduced explanatory variables into their analysis. Amemiya and Boskin used a censored (though they called it "truncated") lognormal distribution to model the duration of welfare dependency. We considered the lognormal distribution as well as the exponential and normal distributions and found that the lognormal provided the best fit to our data. We have continued this line of work in Schmidt and Witte (1979, 1980, 1984) and in this book.

Harris and Moitra (1978) introduced the Weibull distribution (see the section The Weibull Model, Chapter 4) for use in survival analyses of recidivism data. This distribution is a well-known generalization of the exponential distribution and is widely used in survival analyses in biostatistics and operations research. When using the Weibull distribution, one can test to see if the simpler exponential model is appropriate. Harris, Kaylan, and Maltz (1981) compared the fit of the Weibull and three different exponential distributions, and their results indicate that the Weibull model fits their data better than any of the exponential models. Their mixed exponential model also seems to fit reasonably well.

Cox's proportional hazards model has recently been used to analyze the determinants of recidivism by a variety of researchers, including Barton and Turnbull (1981), Rhodes and Matsuba (1985), Sherman and Berk (1984), and Witte et al. (1982). This model incorporates explanatory variables in a particular parametric (usually linear) form, but it is nonparametric in the sense that no specific distribution is assumed for time until recidivism. As we discuss in Chapters 6 and 9 and as Chaiken and Rolph (1981) have pointed out, nonparametric methods like the proportional hazards model are best regarded as useful in preliminary work designed to select an appropriate parametric method. The reason is simple. Even in large data sets, the frequency of return to crime varies erratically over time, despite the presence of a quite discernible trend in the hazard rate. To analyze this underlying trend properly, the data cry out for some sort of smoothing, and this is precisely what parametric methods provide. In preliminary work, one may well wish to estimate a nonparametric model, as we do. This may be useful for determining which explanatory variables are important and as a basis for assessing the adequacy of various parametric models. However, we are firmly convinced, on the basis of our work, that parametric models fit recidivism data better and provide more accurate predictions than nonparametric models do.

Our work draws many insights from the literature reviewed earlier and extends it in a number of directions. First, we consider and compare the adequacy of many different models. We are careful to include in our selection the models previously used in the literature (i.e., the exponential, lognormal, Weibull, and proportional hazards models). However, we do not limit ourselves to these models. We evaluate each model that we consider on the basis of its predictive ability. It is essential to emphasize that although our best models are quite good, our worst models are quite bad. No one should consider using a survival model without being willing to conduct tests of its adequacy. We believe that one of the major contributions of our work is our thorough evaluation of a large number of survival models for use with recidivism data.[23]

Second, we compare in considerable detail the predictive ability of models that do and do not explicitly incorporate explanatory variables, as well as the possible uses of both kinds of models. We believe that this is an important contribution as the literature that does not use explanatory variables (e.g., the work of Stollmack and Harris and of Maltz and his colleagues) and the literature that does (e.g., the work of Schmidt and Witte and the work that uses the proportional hazards model) have largely developed separately. We find uses for both types of models. The models that do not use explanatory variables predict quite well for random samples of the population, whereas models with explanatory variables can allow one to gain insights into the causes of crime, make individual predictions, and predict for nonrandom samples.

Finally, we evaluate the usefulness of split population models and extend these models to allow separate sets of explanatory variables to explain the

---

[23] Witte and Schmidt (1977), Harris et al. (1981), and Maltz (1984) provide evaluations of a much smaller range of models.

probability of recidivism and the timing of recidivism for those who do return to crime. We believe this extension will prove very useful as more people come to estimate "career criminal" models on data for offenders and for general population groups.

Preview of Coming Attractions

In the next chapter, we describe the data we use to estimate our models. The data consist of information on 1978 and 1980 cohorts of releasees from North Carolina's state prisons. Chapter 3 provides a brief description of the statistical methodology used in the book and is recommended reading for anyone wishing to understand the material that follows. For those not interested in technical details, it is important to glean from this chapter at least an understanding of basic concepts, such as the density function, the cumulative distribution function, and the hazard rate.

Chapter 4 contains our analysis of simple parametric and nonparametric models that do not include explanatory variables. These models follow in the tradition of Stollmack and Harris (1974) but consider a much broader range of models than were considered previously. Furthermore, we evaluate the ability of the alternative models to predict for a validation sample from the same release cohort as the estimation sample and for a validation sample from a different release cohort. This is one of the few instances in which researchers have sought to check the predictive accuracy of models with data for years of release other than that used to estimate the models. Such research has been called for by Farrington and Tarling (1985) and has been carried out previously by Gottfredson and Gottfredson (1985).

In Chapter 5, we consider "split population" models of the type introduced by Maltz and McCleary (1977). We find that these models predict remarkably more accurately than the simple models of Chapter 4.

Chapter 6 contains our estimates of the proportional hazards model. This is the first model we consider that contains explanatory variables. It is used as a benchmark to compare the predictive accuracy of our parametric models with explanatory variables and as a preliminary basis for choosing which explanatory variables to include in these models.

In Chapter 7, we consider parametric models with explanatory variables. We find that our parametric models predict more accurately than Cox's proportional hazards model. We also extend the split population model to allow separate processes (and sets of explanatory variables) to determine the probability that an individual will ultimately return to prison and the timing of return for those who will ultimately return. We find that a logit lognormal model, in which the probability of eventual recidivism follows a logit model and the timing of return follows a lognormal distribution, best fits our data. It is this work that will be of most interest to those wishing to estimate a career criminal model using data for general population groups.

In Chapter 8, we turn our attention from prediction for random samples of releasees to prediction for nonrandom samples and individuals. This chapter should be of interest to anyone seeking to use prediction models in evaluation research or criminal justice decision-making.

Finally, Chapter 9 contains our summary and conclusions.

2
Data

The Nature of the Data

The data used in this research project consist of information on two cohorts of releasees from the North Carolina prison system. The first cohort consists of all individuals released from North Carolina prisons from July 1, 1977 through June 30, 1978. There were 9,457 such individuals. The second cohort consists of the 9,679 individuals released from North Carolina prisons from July 1, 1979 through June 30, 1980.[1] Note that these data sets are far larger, more representative, and more timely than is usual in criminal justice research.

We will treat the information on these two cohorts as separate data sets, which we will call the *1978 data set* and the *1980 data set*, respectively. These two data sets will be analyzed in essentially parallel ways. The 1978 and 1980 cohorts differ in their post-release behavior, and one of the purposes of this study is to see whether this difference can be explained by differences in observed demographic characteristics or pre-release behavior between the two cohorts.

The use of two different cohorts allows us to check how well our models are likely to stand up if they are used to predict recidivism of future release cohorts. We believe that our use of two large release cohorts is an important and innovative aspect of our work.

For each cohort, a few observations were obviously defective and had to be discarded. Purely by coincidence, the number of discarded observations was the same for each cohort; 130. In almost all cases, the defect in the data leading to elimination of the observation was that the individual was not in fact released from prison during the time period which defined the

---

[1] We have previously analyzed a cohort consisting of the 4,881 individuals released from prison in North Carolina in the first 6 months of 1975 (Schmidt & Witte, 1978). See Schmidt and Witte (1984, appendix B) for a description of this data set.

data set.[2] It is important to note that the number of defective cases was only slightly more than one percent of the original number of cases. This is a very low discard rate for release cohort data and attests to the high quality of the North Carolina record-keeping system. This system was originally developed in the 1960s and has been improved greatly over time. As noted by Farrington and Tarling (1985) and Gottfredson and Gottfredson (1985), better data quality is central to the improvement of prediction research. While the North Carolina data are not ideal, they are among the best that we are aware of for modeling time until recidivism for prison releasees.

After deletion of these 130 observations from each data set, we are left with 9,327 observations for 1978 and 9,549 observations for 1980. We will refer to these sets of observations as the *basic samples* (for 1978 and 1980, respectively).

In each of the two basic samples, many observations lacked information on one or more variables that we used in our analyses. In the 1978 basic sample, only 4,618 observations contained information on all variables of interest; the other 4,709 observations lacked some information. We will refer to these two subsamples as the *complete data sample* and the *missing data sample*, respectively. The vast majority of the observations in the missing data sample lack information on alcohol or drug abuse, which turns out to be a very significant predictor of post-release criminality; 4,287 of the 4,709 observations in the missing data sample lack this information. The other variables for which information is sometimes missing are marital status, number of previous incarcerations, and years of schooling. The numbers of observations lacking information on these variables are 709, 478, and 116, respectively.

For the 1980 basic sample, there are fewer incomplete observations. The complete data sample contains 5,739 observations, and the missing data sample contains 3,810. Again, most of the incomplete observations (3,396) lack information on alcohol or drug abuse. The smaller percentage of incomplete observations in the 1980 cohort is largely a reflection of a continuing increase over time in the correctness and completeness of the North Carolina Department of Correction's records. However, it is also a reflection of a change in the nature of the release cohort. The type of releasee whose record is most likely to lack information is a short-term misdemeanant, whose social history may not have been taken before release. This type of individual has been diverted increasingly from the

[2] For the 1978 cohort, 126 individuals turned out to have release dates outside the time period (July 1, 1977–June 30, 1978) that defined the cohort. Six individuals had lengths of time until recidivism that were physically impossible; one individual had a value of time served for the previous offense that exceeded his age; and one individual had only an asterisk in his record for month of release. For the 1980 cohort, the reasons for deletions were similar.

prison system in North Carolina and is therefore less common in the 1980 cohort than in the 1978 cohort.

The 1978 and 1980 complete samples were each split randomly into an *estimation sample*[3] and a *validation sample*. For 1978, there are 1,540 observations in the estimation sample and 3,078 observations in the validation sample; for 1980, the corresponding sample sizes are 1,435 and 4,304. For each cohort, we fit our statistical models to the estimation sample and then used the validation sample to check the predictive accuracy of the models. This procedure reflects the generally accepted view that the predictive accuracy of a model can be checked validly only with data not used to estimate the model.

It should be noted that we checked the predictive accuracy of our models for all four of our samples (the 1978 estimation sample, the 1978 validation sample, the 1980 estimation sample, and the 1980 validation sample). This represents a much more thorough testing of the predictive ability of models of recidivism than has occurred in the past. Many prediction studies (e.g., Glueck & Glueck, 1950; Greenwood, 1982) check the predictive power of their models only by considering how well the models predict for the sample used to estimate the model (the estimation sample, in our terminology). Others (e.g., Farrington, 1985; Schmidt & Witte, 1978, 1984) test the predictive power of their model by splitting their data randomly into estimation and validation samples and predicting for the randomly selected validation sample. Occasionally (e.g., Gottfredson & Gottfredson 1985), researchers have used a data set for 1 year to estimate a model and then used the model to predict for a data set for a later year. We combine these various approaches and thus provide an unusually complete evaluation of our models.

The variables used in our analyses will be defined in the following section. Comparisons of the various samples defined above will be given in the section Comparisons of Subsamples.

Definitions of Variables

We will now define the variables used in our study. We distinguish the outcome (dependent or criterion) variables from the explanatory (independent) variables. Basically, the outcome variables are an indicator of whether the individual returned to prison within the follow-up period and the length of time until return for those individuals who did return; the explanatory variables are demographic characteristics and measures of the past criminal and correctional histories of the individuals.

[3] The *estimation sample* will also be called the *analysis sample*; we will use these two terms interchangeably.

To be more specific, recall that individuals in the 1978 data set were released from prison from July 1977 through June 1978, and that individuals in the 1980 data set were released from prison from July 1979 through June 1980. The sentence from which they were released will be called the *sample sentence*, and the corresponding conviction, which resulted in the sample sentence, will be called the *sample conviction*. All explanatory variables are defined either at the time of entry or at the time of release (from the sample sentence). The outcome variables were defined as the result of a search of North Carolina Department of Correction records in April 1984. Thus the follow-up period ranged from 46 to 57 months for the 1980 data set and from 70 to 81 months for the 1978 data set. These follow-up periods are quite long for a study of recidivism, and we believe that this is an important strength of our study. Most studies follow releasees for 3 years or less. There are important advantages to having long follow-ups when estimating survival models. First, the correct distribution for time until recidivism is easier to discover if we observe recidivism rates over a longer period of time. Second, the censoring problem (correct treatment of individuals who have not yet returned to prison at the end of the follow-up) is less serious the longer the follow-up is, as fewer individuals are censored.

We define the following outcome variables for each individual:

FOLLOW = the length of the follow-up period, in months.

RECID = a dummy (indicator) variable equal to one if the individual returned to a North Carolina prison during the follow-up period and equal to zero otherwise.

TIME = the length of time from release from prison until return to prison, rounded to the nearest month, for individuals for whom RECID = 1. TIME is undefined for individuals for whom RECID = 0.

We now define the following explanatory variables for each individual:

TSERVD = the time served (in months) for the sample sentence.

AGE = age (in months) at time of release.

PRIORS = the number of previous incarcerations, not including the sample sentence, at the time of entry into the prison system for the sample sentence.

RULE = the number of prison rule violations reported during the sample sentence.

SCHOOL = the number of years of formal schooling completed at the time of entry into the prison system for the sample sentence.

WHITE = a dummy variable equal to zero if the individual is black and equal to one otherwise.[4]

[4] Basically, WHITE equals one for whites and zero for blacks. However, the North Carolina prison population does contain a small number of Native Americans, Hispanics, Orientals, and individuals of "other" race. They are treated as whites by this definition.

MALE = a dummy variable equal to one if the individual is male and equal to zero if female.
ALCHY = a dummy variable equal to one if the individual's record indicates a serious problem with alcohol (before entry into the prison system) and equal to zero otherwise.
JUNKY = a dummy variable equal to one if the individual's record indicates use of hard drugs (before entry into the prison system) and equal to zero otherwise.
MARRIED = a dummy variable equal to one if the individual was married at the time of entry into prison for the sample sentence and equal to zero otherwise.
SUPER = a dummy variable equal to one if the individual's release from the sample sentence was supervised (e.g., parole) and equal to zero otherwise.
WORKREL = a dummy variable equal to one if the individual participated in the North Carolina prisoner work release program during the sample sentence and equal to zero otherwise.
FELON = a dummy variable equal to one if the sample sentence was for a felony and equal to zero if it was for a misdemeanor.
PERSON = a dummy variable equal to one if the sample sentence was for a crime against a person and equal to zero otherwise.
PROPTY = a dummy variable equal to one if the sample sentence was for a crime against property and equal to zero otherwise.[5]

Comparisons of Subsamples

Table 2.1 gives a complete listing of the distribution of TIME for the 1978 analysis and validation samples. For each number of months (N) from zero through the maximum follow-up period of 81, this table lists the number of individuals at risk at the beginning of the month, the number of individuals who return to prison during the month, and the number of individuals censored (in the sense that the follow-up period ends without the individual having returned to prison) during the month.[6] Table 2.2 provides the same information for the 1980 analysis and validation samples.

The timing of recidivism seen in Tables 2.1 and 2.2 has a number of

[5] If the sample sentence resulted from several convictions, the variables FELON, PERSON, and PROPTY are defined on the basis of the conviction resulting in the longest sentence. Note also that some convictions are for crimes not classified as crimes against a person or crimes against property, so that PERSON and PROPTY do contain independent information. The categorization of offenses as PERSON, PROPTY, or "other" is that of Witte (1975).

[6] Note that the way in which TIME is rounded to the nearest month means that $N = 0$ corresponds to the first 15 days after release, $N = 1$ corresponds to the month thereafter, and so forth.

TABLE 2.1. Data summary, 1978.

	Analysis sample			Validation sample		
N	At risk	Returned	Censored	At risk	Returned	Censored
0	1,540	1	0	3,078	0	0
1	1,539	7	0	3,078	16	0
2	1,532	15	0	3,062	14	0
3	1,517	14	0	3,048	29	0
4	1,503	13	0	3,019	35	0
5	1,490	16	0	2,984	35	0
6	1,474	18	0	2,949	40	0
7	1,456	19	0	2,909	43	0
8	1,437	16	0	2,866	41	0
9	1,421	18	0	2,825	36	0
10	1,403	22	0	2,789	39	0
11	1,381	12	0	2,750	37	0
12	1,369	17	0	2,713	38	0
13	1,352	15	0	2,675	39	0
14	1,337	16	0	2,636	24	0
15	1,321	24	0	2,612	25	0
16	1,297	13	0	2,587	36	0
17	1,284	9	0	2,551	22	0
18	1,275	17	0	2,529	24	0
19	1,258	10	0	2,505	22	0
20	1,248	8	0	2,483	21	0
21	1,240	14	0	2,462	18	0
22	1,226	7	0	2,444	19	0
23	1,219	17	0	2,425	17	0
24	1,202	12	0	2,403	21	0
25	1,190	14	0	2,387	22	0
26	1,176	8	0	2,365	22	0
27	1,168	11	0	2,343	19	0
28	1,157	9	0	2,324	18	0
29	1,148	8	0	2,306	21	0
30	1,140	7	0	2,285	13	0
31	1,133	6	0	2,272	7	0
32	1,127	6	0	2,265	8	0
33	1,121	6	0	2,257	13	0
34	1,115	4	0	2,244	14	0
35	1,111	6	0	2,230	14	0
36	1,105	6	0	2,216	12	0
37	1,099	6	0	2,204	14	0
38	1,093	4	0	2,190	9	0
39	1,089	4	0	2,181	10	0
40	1,085	2	0	2,171	9	0
41	1,083	8	0	2,162	11	0
42	1,075	5	0	2,151	6	0
43	1,070	5	0	2,145	13	0
44	1,065	4	0	2,132	8	0
45	1,061	4	0	2,124	11	0
46	1,057	7	0	2,113	11	0
47	1,050	4	0	2,102	6	0
48	1,046	1	0	2,096	12	0

TABLE 2.1. *Continued.*

	Analysis sample			Validation sample		
N	At risk	Returned	Censored	At risk	Returned	Censored
49	1,045	5	0	2,084	7	0
50	1,040	6	0	2,077	10	0
51	1,034	3	0	2,067	3	0
52	1,031	2	0	2,064	8	0
53	1,029	8	0	2,056	5	0
54	1,021	3	0	2,051	6	0
55	1,018	5	0	2,045	4	0
56	1,013	2	0	2,041	9	0
57	1,011	4	0	2,032	8	0
58	1,007	1	0	2,024	6	0
59	1,006	5	0	2,018	5	0
60	1,001	3	0	2,013	7	0
61	998	0	0	2,006	10	0
62	998	3	0	1,996	7	0
63	995	2	0	1,989	7	0
64	993	1	0	1,982	6	0
65	992	2	0	1,976	8	0
66	990	3	0	1,968	7	0
67	987	3	0	1,961	5	0
68	984	4	0	1,956	4	0
69	980	2	0	1,952	5	0
70	978	2	110	1,947	4	196
71	966	2	102	1,747	2	180
72	762	1	90	1,565	3	185
73	671	1	115	1,377	3	217
74	555	1	78	1,157	6	168
75	476	0	46	983	1	99
76	430	0	111	883	0	216
77	319	1	66	667	1	132
78	252	0	55	534	0	121
79	197	0	66	413	0	133
80	131	0	77	280	0	161
81	54	0	54	119	0	119

TABLE 2.2. Data summary, 1980.

	Analysis sample			Validation sample		
N	At risk	Returned	Censored	At risk	Returned	Censored
0	1,435	1	0	4,304	6	0
1	1,434	6	0	4,298	14	0
2	1,428	11	0	4,284	41	0
3	1,417	19	0	4,243	67	0
4	1,398	20	0	4,176	71	0
5	1,378	24	0	4,105	76	0
6	1,354	29	0	4,029	66	0
7	1,325	24	0	3,963	62	0

TABLE 2.2. *Continued.*

	Analysis sample			Validation sample		
N	At risk	Returned	Censored	At risk	Returned	Censored
8	1,301	16	0	3,901	75	0
9	1,285	17	0	3,826	65	0
10	1,268	22	0	3,761	66	0
11	1,246	17	0	3,695	66	0
12	1,229	15	0	3,629	62	0
13	1,214	15	0	3,567	49	0
14	1,199	16	0	3,518	48	0
15	1,183	11	0	3,470	49	0
16	1,172	16	0	3,421	39	0
17	1,156	15	0	3,382	42	0
18	1,141	10	0	3,340	42	0
19	1,131	16	0	3,298	27	0
20	1,115	13	0	3,271	40	0
21	1,102	11	0	3,231	35	0
22	1,091	5	0	3,196	19	0
23	1,086	4	0	3,177	30	0
24	1,082	7	0	3,147	23	0
25	1,075	4	0	3,124	32	0
26	1,071	12	0	3,092	25	0
27	1,059	9	0	3,067	28	0
28	1,050	4	0	3,039	18	0
29	1,046	9	0	3,021	20	0
30	1,037	10	0	3,001	17	0
31	1,027	9	0	2,984	19	0
32	1,018	8	0	2,965	29	0
33	1,010	11	0	2,936	18	0
34	999	11	0	2,918	22	0
35	988	5	0	2,896	28	0
36	983	9	0	2,868	19	0
37	974	11	0	2,849	10	0
38	963	5	0	2,839	14	0
39	958	6	0	2,825	17	0
40	952	2	0	2,808	15	0
41	950	8	0	2,793	14	0
42	942	2	0	2,779	11	0
43	940	7	0	2,768	15	0
44	933	7	0	2,753	9	0
45	926	6	0	2,744	10	0
46	920	0	93	2,734	12	294
47	827	2	75	2,428	8	213
48	750	1	58	2,207	5	214
49	691	2	90	1,988	6	191
50	599	2	76	1,791	5	199
51	521	3	64	1,587	3	174
52	454	0	84	1,410	3	273
53	370	1	78	1,134	1	250
54	291	4	72	883	1	256
55	215	0	71	626	0	201
56	144	0	72	425	1	225
57	72	0	72	199	0	199

interesting aspects which are important to consider when selecting a statistical model. These are perhaps best seen by considering the probability that an individual will return to prison during a given month, assuming survival up to the beginning of that month; this is the hazard rate. Note that the hazard rate rises during the early months after release and then falls rapidly. These trends are very clear in both Tables 2.1 and 2.2, despite considerable random fluctuations (noise) around the trend. For example, consider the hazard rate for the 1978 analysis sample. It begins at the very low level of .001 (that is, one-tenth of 1%) for the first 15 days after release and then rises in a jagged but clear fashion to a peak of .018 at 15 months after release. It then falls rapidly to essentially zero at the end of the follow-up period. The hazard rate for the 1980 analysis sample has the same general pattern, but the peak hazard rate is higher (.021 versus .018) and occurs earlier (after 6 months instead of 15). The hazard rate also declines more rapidly in the 1980 sample.

This pattern for the hazard rate is not commonly found in applications of survival analysis in biostatistics or operations research, and therefore we should not expect the straightforward adoption of models used in those areas to be very successful. As noted in the section Previous Use of Survival Analysis in Justice Research (Chapter 1), most previous applications of survival analysis in justice research have simply adopted models from those literatures. Although we do estimate previously used models, as a matter of comparison with the models which we believe are more appropriate, we basically adopt the strategy of searching the statistical literature to find distributions with the type of behavior of the hazard rate that is found in our data.

It is interesting to speculate as to why the hazard rate in data on recidivism has the pattern which it does. Carr-Hill and Carr-Hill (1972) point out that the functioning of the criminal justice system ensures that we will not observe reconviction or return to prison until some time after the actual criminal offense has occurred. Thus, the hazard rate for reconviction or return to prison should indeed start at a low level and increase for the first few months after release.

The time that it takes for the criminal justice system to process cases can perhaps explain why the hazard rate for our 1980 data does not peak until 6 months after release. However, it is implausible that the time lag explains the peak at 15 months after release in the 1978 data. It may be that there really is a period of time after release in which many releasees try to "go straight," and they return to crime only after being disappointed in this attempt.

The eventual decrease in the hazard rate is common to data on recidivism (and in many other fields of application) and may occur for either or both of two reasons. First, behavior at the individual level may indeed change with elapsed time since release. For example, the rate of commission of crimes may decrease, or an individual may become more adept at escaping detection. Second, if individuals differ in their rates of criminality (as they almost certainly do) and therefore in their likelihood of recidivism, we should expect that most of the recidivists in the early months after release are individuals with a high propensity for recidivism. As time passes, the surviving release cohort will be made up more and more of individuals with a low propensity for recidivism, and thus the hazard rate of the surviving group should fall.

Table 2.3 gives the mean values of the variables defined in the last section, for various subsamples of the 1978 data set, and Table 2.4 does the same for the 1980 data set. For each variable, the mean value is given for the basic sample, the missing data sample, the complete data sample, the analysis sample, and the validation sample. For those variables that take on a continuous range of values (for example, AGE), the mean value has an obvious interpretation. For those variables that are dummy (indicator) variables (for example, MALE = one for males and zero for females), the mean value is the proportion of the sample which has the characteristic indicated.

TABLE 2.3. Means of variables, 1978 data.

Variable	Basic sample[a]	Missing data[b]	Complete data[c]	Analysis[d]	Validation[e]	Test, M = C	Test, A = V
FOLLOW	75.270	75.580	74.960	74.890	75.000	8.46	−1.04
RECID	.381	.395	.373	.370	.374	2.23	−.25
TIME	24.580	24.920	24.200	23.880	24.360	1.14	−.51
TSERVD	19.750	20.040	19.460	18.800	19.790	1.04	−1.50
AGE	351.800	359.900	343.500	346.100	342.200	6.24	1.05
PRIORS	1.507	1.664	1.364	1.377	1.358	4.47	.22
RULE	1.263	1.313	1.211	1.131	1.250	1.73	−1.51
SCHOOL	9.551	9.427	9.675	9.724	9.650	−4.96	.97
WHITE	.513	.499	.518	.509	.522	1.84	−.85
MALE	.959	.958	.941	.938	.943	3.54	−.66
ALCHY	.207	.275	.201	.210	.196	3.61	1.10
JUNKY	.277	.453	.261	.239	.272	8.41	−2.42
MARRIED	.301	.344	.264	.256	.268	8.05	−.92
SUPER	.684	.660	.696	.698	.696	3.80	.17
WORKREL	.409	.349	.462	.455	.465	11.10	−.69
FELON	.275	.227	.318	.312	.321	9.85	−.62
PERSON	.052	.047	.055	.060	.053	1.81	.49
PROPTY	.224	.190	.255	.251	.257	6.43	−.48

[a] N = 9,327 except: TIME, 3,582; PRIORS, 8,849; SCHOOL, 9,211; ALCHY, JUNKY, 5,040; MARRIED, 8,618.

[b] N = 4,709 except: TIME, 1,861; PRIORS, 4,231; SCHOOL, 4,593; ALCHY, JUNKY, 422; MARRIED, 4,000.

[c] N = 4,618 except: TIME, 1,721.

[d] N = 1,540 except: TIME, 570.

[e] N = 3,078 except: TIME, 1,151.

TABLE 2.4. Means of variables, 1980 data.

Variable	Basic sample[a]	Missing data[b]	Complete data[c]	Analysis[d]	Validation[e]	Test, M = C	Test, A = V
FOLLOW	51.420	51.400	51.430	51.420	51.430	−.32	−.09
RECID	.369	.361	.374	.369	.375	1.23	−.40
TIME	17.850	17.950	17.790	18.860	17.430	.38	2.26
TSERVD	18.710	17.830	19.300	19.520	19.230	−2.83	.43
AGE	350.100	363.500	341.100	339.000	341.900	8.71	−.81
PRIORS	1.432	1.597	1.347	1.392	1.332	3.84	.70
RULE	1.538	1.623	1.481	1.452	1.491	1.75	−.40
SCHOOL	9.626	9.623	9.628	9.647	9.622	−.08	.35
WHITE	.505	.495	.511	.510	.511	2.02	.00
MALE	.934	.918	.944	.946	.944	5.02	.36
ALCHY	.363	.406	.359	.357	.360	1.90	−.25
JUNKY	.202	.203	.202	.218	.196	.00	1.78
MARRIED	.257	.296	.234	.234	.233	6.60	.00
SUPER	.775	.718	.812	.801	.816	7.65	−1.21
WORKREL	.406	.370	.430	.433	.429	5.82	.30
FELON	.385	.336	.417	.431	.413	8.01	1.17
PERSON	.113	.113	.112	.113	.112	.10	.09
PROPTY	.424	.397	.442	.447	.440	4.36	.22

[a] N = 9,549 except: TIME, 3,522; PRIORS, 8,680; SCHOOL, 9,452; ALCHY, JUNKY, 6,153; MARRIED, 9,235.
[b] N = 3,810 except: TIME, 1,377; PRIORS, 2,941; SCHOOL, 3,713; ALCHY, JUNKY, 414; MARRIED, 3,496.
[c] N = 5,739 except: TIME, 2,145.
[d] N = 1,435 except: TIME, 530.
[e] N = 4,304 except: TIME, 1,615.

The column titled "Test, M = C" gives the *t*-statistics used to test the statistical significance of the differences in the mean values of the variables in the missing data sample and the complete data sample. Similarly, the column titled "Test, A = V" gives the *t*-statistics used to test the significance of the differences in the mean values of the variables between the analysis sample and the validation sample. Given the large number of observations in our samples, these test statistics should be compared to the critical values of the standard normal distribution; for example, a value in excess of 1.96 in absolute value is significant at the 5% level.

Since the analysis and validation samples are chosen as *random* subsamples of the complete data sample, significant differences between the analysis and validation samples arise only by chance. For the most part, the differences we find are as small as would be expected. In each cohort, one variable's mean value is significantly different at the 5% level in the analysis and validation samples: JUNKY in the 1978 data and TIME in the 1980 data. Given 18 such differences (for each cohort), it is certainly not surprising that, by chance, one should be significant at the 5% level. However, it is unfortunate that one such large difference should be in the dependent variable (TIME) which we will analyze. As we will see later, virtually all of our models that are fit to the 1980 analysis sample underpredict the rate of recidivism in the 1980 validation sample. This is presumably to be expected, given the significant difference in the mean values of TIME in the two samples.

On the other hand, the division of the basic sample into the missing data and complete data samples is certainly *not* random, and we should anticipate differences between these two samples. The main reason why an individual's record lacks information on one or more variables is that a social history was not taken upon admission to prison for the sample sentence. Such an omission would be more likely for a short-term misdemeanant, whose stay in the prison system was expected to be brief, than for an individual with a longer sentence.

This expectation is only partly born out in the data. Individuals with missing data are indeed more likely to be misdemeanants than are individuals with complete data, but only in the 1980 cohort is their average time served shorter. Other significant differences also occur. For example, in both cohorts, individuals with missing data are older, more often black, and more likely to be married; they have more prior incarcerations; their sample sentence is less likely to be for a crime against property; and they are less likely to be released on supervision or to have participated in the work release program. Individuals with missing data also appear more likely to be alcoholics, though this is not clear because so many of the individuals with missing data are missing information on exactly this variable (ALCHY). Finally, it is worth noting that there is no consistent significant difference in *outcome* variables between the missing data and complete data samples.

Comparing Table 2.3 with Table 2.4 reveals some considerable differences between the 1978 and 1980 release cohorts. Perhaps the most striking is in the nature of the offense for which the releasees were last imprisoned, which tends to be much more serious in the 1980 cohort than in the 1978 cohort. This reflects a nationwide trend to incarcerate increasingly the more serious offenders. An individual released in 1980 is about twice as likely to have been imprisoned for a crime against a person or a crime against property (the two classifications that include most of the more serious crimes) than an individual released in 1978, and about 50% more likely to have been imprisoned for a felony. This is obviously consistent with the notion that, over time, increasingly severe space constraints have caused imprisonment to be reserved for more serious offenders. An individual released in 1980 is also almost twice as likely to be classified as having a serious problem with alcohol than is an individual released in 1978. On the other hand, a 1980 releasee is less likely to be identified as a user of hard drugs, which is hard to explain.

A less obvious difference is that the rate of recidivism is significantly higher in the 1980 release cohort than in the 1978 cohort. This is not really visible in Tables 2.3 and 2.4, because differences in recidivism rates reported there are confounded by the considerable difference in the average follow-up period. Although the overall proportion of recidivists is slightly *lower* in the 1980 cohort, this is entirely due to the fact that the follow-up period is two years shorter than for the 1978 cohort. If we standardize the follow-up period, the higher recidivism rate in the 1980 cohort becomes apparent. For example, if we pick a follow-up period of 46 months, which is the minimum for individuals in either cohort, the recidivism rate is .359 for the 1980 cohort and only .324 for the 1978 cohort. Similar differences exist for follow-up periods shorter than 46 months (but which are held the same for the two cohorts).

An interesting question that this raises is whether the difference in recidivism rates between the two cohorts can be accounted for in terms of differences in observed characteristics of the releasees. In Chapter 8, we report that it can. Although models fit to the 1978 data tend to under-predict the recidivism experience in the 1980 data, the best models making use of individual characteristics as explanatory variables predict quite accurately for both years. Thus we have some evidence that the change in behavior is due to the changing characteristics of the prison population. North Carolina is apparently incarcerating offenders who are more likely to commit additional offenses and whose observable characteristics make this outcome predictable.

With this in mind, it is perhaps useful to paint a portrait of the typical releasee in 1978 and 1980. The typical releasee in 1978 was a single male who was approximately equally likely to be white or black, was not addicted to alcohol or drugs, and was convicted of a victimless offense (our "other" category). He was approximately 29 years of age with two prior incarcerations, 10 years of education, and one rule violation while in prison.

The typical 1980 releasee was also most commonly a 29-year-old single male who had 10 years of education, was equally likely to be white or black, and was not addicted to alcohol or drugs. However, he had slightly fewer prior arrests, was almost twice as likely as a 1978 releasee to be convicted of a property offense, and was less well-behaved while in prison. By 1980, the prison system was releasing substantially more property offenders, and they were less able to abide by institutional rules.

3
Survey of Statistical Methodology

Survival Time Models

In this chapter, we will give a brief description of the statistical methodology used in this study. We are interested in formulating and estimating models of the length of time from an individual's release from prison until his or her recidivism; we will use these models to predict the rate of recidivism among other groups of individuals. The details of estimation will be given in the section Estimation of Survival Time Models, and the details of prediction, including assessing the accuracy of the predictions, will be given in the section Predictions Using Survival Time Models. In this first section, we will give a brief, general discussion of the nature of the problem. A more thorough treatment of this topic can be found in Schmidt and Witte (1984, Chapter 6).

From a statistical point of view, the length of time until recidivism is a survival time (or failure time), and the enormous statistical literature on survival times is relevant.[1] While most of that literature deals with biological applications (e.g., survival times of medical patients) or engineering applications (e.g., time until equipment failure), the statistical problems are in some ways analogous in criminological applications such as ours.

However, as noted in Chapter 1, the simple adoption of models from operations research or biostatistics is potentially dangerous for two reasons. First, these models are based on statistical distributions that may not be appropriate for data on recidivism. For example, models based on the exponential distribution imply a constant hazard rate, and models based on the Weibull distribution imply a hazard rate which is either constant, monotonically increasing, or montonically decreasing. In our data, and probably in most other data on recidivism, the hazard rate first

[1] There are several good textbook treatments of the topic, including Cox and Oates (1984), Kalbfleisch and Prentice (1980), and Lawless (1982).

rises and then falls. This behavior of the hazard rate does not seem to be observed in typical applications reported in the statistical literature on survival analysis, and it cannot be accomodated by the standard statistical models developed there. Second, survival models in biostatistics and operations research generally do not consider a wide range of explanatory variables. We believe that it is quite important to consider a wide array of explanatory variables in our analyses and probably in most criminal justice applications of survival models. The reason is that both prior research and criminological theory suggest that criminal activity is determined by a variety of factors, which must be considered explicitly to provide adequate models of recidivism.

An essential feature of survival times is that they are almost always *censored* (i.e., they are not observed for all individuals in the sample). In our case, this occurs because not every member of a release cohort will have returned to prison by the end of the follow-up period. Indeed, despite our fairly long follow-up periods (70–81 months for the 1978 cohort and 46–57 months for the 1980 cohort), approximately 65% of the releasees had not returned to prison by the end of their follow-up period. For these individuals, we have no way of knowing when or if they ultimately will fail. All we know is that their survival time is at least as long as the length of their follow-up period.

When data are censored, it is essential that this is taken into account in estimation. Methods of estimation that do not account for censoring, such as least squares regression analysis or logit and probit analysis, can give severely distorted results when applied to censored data. For example, one might consider avoiding the censoring problem by analyzing the survival times of only those individuals who failed before the end of their follow-up period.[2] This is not a good idea because the individuals who fail are surely very different from those who do not; the sample of failures, therefore, is not representative of the original sample of releasees. We would certainly expect that models fit to samples of individuals who fail would *underpredict* time until recidivism (and therefore would overpredict the rate of recidivism) for entire cohorts of releasees. Similarly, one might consider setting the survival time equal to the length of the follow-up period for those individuals who did not yet fail; again, it is reasonable to assume that models fit to such data would underpredict time until recidivism for a release cohort. However, techniques that take censoring into account in estimation do exist, and when these techniques are used, there is no reason to expect systematic underprediction of time until recidivism. We explore such techniques in this book.

A second obvious feature of time until recidivism is that it is nonnegative. Furthermore, it is likely to have a long and "fat" right tail;

[2] As an example, see Brannas and Eklof (1985).

although many individuals fail quickly, some may continue to fail after quite long periods of time. These are common features of failure times and have led to the use of a variety of probability distributions which also have these features (e.g., lognormal, Weibull, and Pareto). We will employ a number of these distributions in Chapter 4.

Estimation of Survival Time Models

In this section, we will give a general treatment of the estimation of survival time models. The discussion will be of so-called parametric models, in which a particular form of the distribution of survival time is assumed. Nonparametric models will be covered later in Chapters 4 and 6.

To consider the problem of estimation in a general setting, suppose that for a particular population (in our case, a release cohort), the survival time t is assumed to follow a particular distribution that is characterized by a cumulative distribution function, $F(t)$. This distribution function is assumed to be defined for all $t > 0$. Corresponding to the distribution function $F(t)$ are the density $f(t)$ and the hazard rate:

$$h(t) = f(t)/[1 - F(t)].$$

These three functions are equivalent representations of the distribution of survival time, in the sense that, from any one of the three (F, f, or h), the other two functions can be derived. They have well-known interpretations, as follows. The distribution function $F(t)$ gives the proportion of the population that will fail no later than time t; that is, $F(t)$ is the usual recidivism rate for the length of follow-up equal to t. The density $f(t)$ gives the failure rate at time t as a proportion of the entire population. The hazard rate (or conditional failure rate) $h(t)$ gives the failure rate at time t as a proportion of the part of the population that has survived up to time t. Each of these functions will depend on some unkown parameters, say θ, and in some cases will also depend on some characteristics of the individual releasee, say X, so that we might write more accurately $F(t;X,\theta)$, $f(t;X,\theta)$, and $h(t;X,\theta)$. However, this seems unnecessarily cumbersome, and we will write simply $F(t)$, $f(t)$, and $h(t)$.

Suppose now that our data consist of information on a sample of size N from this population and that we index individuals by $i = 1, \ldots, N$. For individual i we observe the following information. First, we know the follow-up time, say T_i; in our data set, this corresponds to the variable FOLLOW, defined in the previous chapter. Second, we know whether the individual returned to prison before the end of the follow-up period. We can express this by a dummy (indicator) variable, say C_i, which equals one if the individual returned to prison and equals zero if he or she did not; in our data set, this corresponds to the variable RECID. Third, for those individuals who did return to prison, we know the failure time t_i, which corresponds to the variable TIME in our data set. Fourth, if individual characteristics are allowed to influence the distribution of survival time, we observe the vector $\mathbf{X}_i$ of such characteristics.

We are now in a position to write the likelihood function. If individual i is a recidivist at time t_i, the appropriate contribution of observation i to the likelihood function is $f(t_i)$, which is just the density of the observed failure time. On the other hand, if individual i is a nonrecidivist with follow-up period of length T_i, the appropriate contribution to the likelihood function for observation i is $1 - F(T_i)$, which is the probability that the individual has not failed by time T_i. For the entire sample of N observations therefore, the likelihood function is

$$L = \prod_{i=1}^{N} f(t_i)^{C_i} [1 - F(T_i)]^{(1-C_i)}, \tag{3.1}$$

where the symbol π represents multiplication. Note that in Equation 3.1 we have $C_i = 1$, and hence $1 - C_i = 0$, for the recidivists, whereas for the nonrecidivists, we have $C_i = 0$, and hence $1 - C_i = 1$. Thus only one of the two types of terms on the right side of Equation 3.1 actually appears: $f(t_i)$ for the recidivists and $1 - F(T_i)$ for the nonrecidivists.

It is equivalent, and often easier, to work with the logarithm of the likelihood function, namely:

$$\ln L = \sum_{i=1}^{N} \{C_i \ln f(t_i) + (1 - C_i) \ln [1 - F(T_i)]\}. \tag{3.2}$$

Indeed, the logarithm of the likelihood function in Equation 3.2 is often simply called the likelihood function, and we will use this terminology.

The likelihood function depends on the unknown parameters (θ) because they enter into the functions f and F. The *maximum likelihood estimator* (MLE) of θ is defined as the value of θ that maximizes the likelihood function in Equation 3.2. Calculation of the maximum likelihood estimator generally requires a numerical maximization of the likelihood function, which can be difficult and expensive when the number of observations is large and especially when the number of parameters (the dimension of θ) is large.

The maximum likelihood estimator of θ is the value that makes the observed outcomes most likely, an intuitively reasonable criterion. In this study, we will rely almost exclusively on maximum likelihood estimators. Maximum likelihood estimators are well known to have desirable properties in large samples; they are consistent, (asymptotically) efficient, and (asymptotically) normally distributed. Our sample sizes are large, so these are comforting properties for our estimators. This discussion also suggests that survival techniques relying on maximum likelihood estimation generally should be applied only to large samples.

To make this discussion more concrete, we will now provide the details for one of the distributions that we will consider in Chapter 4, namely, the exponential distribution. As noted in Chapter 1, this distribution has been widely used for the analysis of recidivism data. The exponential distribution has the density function:

$$f(t) = \theta e^{-\theta t}; \tag{3.3}$$

and the distribution function:

$$F(t) = 1 - e^{-\theta t}, \tag{3.4}$$

where e is the base of natural logarithms. These are defined for $t \geqslant 0$. Thus the likelihood function in Equation 3.2 becomes:

$$\ln L = \sum_{i=1}^{N} \{C_i (\ln \theta - \theta t_i) + (1 - C_i)(-\theta T_i)\}. \tag{3.5}$$

This can be simplified by defining n as the number of recidivists and by defining t_i^* as t_i for the recidivists and T_i for the nonrecidivists. Then Equation 3.5 becomes:

$$\ln L = n \ln \theta - \theta \sum_{i=1}^{N} t_i^*. \tag{3.6}$$

This is maximized by the MLE of θ, which is:

$$n / \Sigma t_i^*. \tag{3.7}$$

(This is an unusual case in that an explicit solution for the MLE is possible.) For large n, the MLE of θ is normally distributed with mean θ and variance θ^2/n. More details and some references can be found in Schmidt and Witte (1984, p. 89).

Predictions Using Survival Time Models

In this section, we discuss the use of (estimated) survival time models to make predictions. A survival time model gives the probability distribution of the time until recidivism for each individual in some population. This means that we can make probabilistic statements about outcomes for particular individuals. More interesting, however, is that we can make predictions of the outcomes for groups of individuals. For example, if the survival time model implies that the probability of return within 24 months is .15, and we have a release cohort of 1,000 individuals, we can predict that 150 of them should return to prison within 24 months. Furthermore, we can make the usual type of statistical confidence statements reflecting the likely variability of the number of returnees, so that 24 months later, we can say whether the actual number of returnees is or is not *significantly* different (in the statistical sense) from 150. For example, in the hypothetical case just discussed, the model implies a probability of .95 that the number of returnees will be between 125 and 175, and the actual number of returnees is significantly different (at the 5% confidence level) from the predicted number of 150 if it is not in the range between 125 and 175.

The types of predictions that we deal with here may be of practical use. For example, they may be used in evaluating correctional programs, as discussed in Schmidt and Witte (1978, 1979, and 1984, Chapter 8). However, in this study, we are primarily interested in making predictions to test the adequacy of our models. A model that accurately represents the probability distribution of time until recidivism should predict accurately, and we will test this.

In our particular analyses, we will be using models estimated with data from the 1978 and 1980 analysis samples to make predictions for the 1978 and 1980 validation samples. There are 3,078 observations (individuals) in the 1978 validation sample and 4,304 observations in the 1980 validation sample. The numbers of observations are large enough that we are comfortable in relying on large-sample (asymptotic) distributions for the several test statistics that we will define shortly.

To make the following discussion concrete, we refer to Table 3.1. It gives the actual outcomes in the 1978 validation sample, the outcomes predicted by an exponential model (as described at the end of the previous section) fit to the 1978 estimation sample, and various test statistics that we can use to test the significance of the differences between the actual and the predicted outcomes. In later chapters, we will present a number of such tables for different samples and different models, all in more or less the same format.

To interpret Table 3.1, note the first column, headed by N. The entries range from zero through 70, representing months after release. For example, the row corresponding to $N = 30$ gives the results for predictions of outcomes 30 months after release. The upper range, 70 months, is the minimum follow-up time for individuals in the 1978 validation sample. After 70 months, we encounter censoring, so the actual outcomes become uncertain. Similarly, for 1980, we make predictions for zero through 46 months after release, as every individual in the 1980 validation sample has a follow-up period of at least 46 months.

The second column, headed Predicted cdf, gives the cumulative distribution function (cdf) implied by the model. It therefore gives the proportion of the sample that the model predicts should have returned to prison after a given number of months. This is the recidivism rate, which is central to much of criminological analysis. For example, the entry in the row corresponding to 30 months is .183 because the exponential model predicts that 18.3% of the release cohort should have failed within 30 months. More precisely, given that we have rounded the data to the nearest month, this is the proportion of the cohort which the model predicts should have failed within 30.5 months. It is calculated for the exponential model as:

TABLE 3.1. Predicted versus actual recidivism rates for 1978 validation sample using exponential model fit to 1978 analysis sample.

N	Predicted cdf	cdf	t	Predicted density	Density	t	Predicted hazard	Hazard	t	χ^2	df
0	.003	.000	−3.19	.003	.000	−3.19	.003	.000	−3.19	10.2	1
1	.010	.005	−2.62	.007	.005	−.94	.007	.005	−.95	11.1	2
2	.016	.010	−2.90	.007	.005	−1.36	.007	.005	−1.38	13.0	3
3	.023	.019	−1.38	.006	.009	2.03	.007	.010	2.00	17.0	4
4	.029	.031	.40	.006	.011	3.42	.007	.012	3.40	28.5	5
5	.036	.042	1.85	.006	.011	3.46	.007	.012	3.47	40.6	6
6	.042	.055	3.55	.006	.013	4.64	.007	.014	4.68	62.5	7
7	.048	.069	5.30	.006	.014	5.36	.007	.015	5.46	92.3	8
8	.055	.082	6.72	.006	.013	4.95	.007	.014	5.11	118.4	9
9	.061	.094	7.66	.006	.012	3.85	.007	.013	4.04	134.7	10
10	.067	.107	8.76	.006	.013	4.59	.007	.014	4.83	158.0	11
11	.073	.119	9.66	.006	.012	4.17	.007	.013	4.45	177.8	12
12	.079	.131	10.59	.006	.012	4.44	.007	.014	4.77	200.6	13
13	.085	.144	11.56	.006	.013	4.72	.007	.015	5.11	226.7	14
14	.091	.151	11.55	.006	.008	1.27	.007	.009	1.60	229.2	15
15	.097	.160	11.62	.006	.008	1.54	.007	.010	1.88	232.0	16
16	.103	.171	12.37	.006	.012	4.15	.007	.014	4.61	254.0	17
17	.109	.178	12.29	.006	.007	.90	.007	.009	1.27	255.6	18
18	.115	.186	12.35	.006	.008	1.40	.007	.009	1.80	258.8	19
19	.121	.193	12.31	.006	.007	.96	.007	.009	1.36	260.7	20
20	.127	.200	12.24	.006	.007	.75	.007	.008	1.15	262.0	21
21	.133	.206	12.02	.006	.006	.07	.007	.007	.44	262.2	22
22	.138	.212	11.88	.006	.006	.34	.007	.008	.72	262.7	23
23	.144	.218	11.66	.006	.006	−.12	.007	.007	.26	262.8	24
24	.150	.224	11.66	.006	.007	.87	.007	.009	1.29	264.4	25
25	.155	.232	11.72	.006	.007	1.15	.007	.009	1.59	267.0	26
26	.161	.239	11.79	.006	.007	1.18	.007	.009	1.63	269.6	27
27	.166	.245	11.73	.005	.006	.48	.007	.008	.91	270.4	28
28	.172	.251	11.63	.005	.006	.27	.007	.008	.69	270.9	29
29	.177	.258	11.69	.005	.007	1.03	.007	.009	1.49	273.1	30
30	.183	.262	11.38	.005	.004	−.91	.007	.006	−.53	273.4	31
31	.188	.264	10.81	.005	.002	−2.36	.007	.003	−2.07	277.7	32
32	.193	.267	10.31	.005	.003	−2.09	.007	.004	−1.80	280.9	33
33	.199	.271	10.05	.005	.004	−.83	.007	.006	−.49	281.2	34

34	.204	.276	9.85	.005	.005	−.56	.007	.006	−.21	281.2	35
35	.209	.280	9.66	.005	.005	−.54	.007	.006	−.18	281.2	36
36	.214	.284	9.40	.005	.004	−1.01	.007	.005	−.68	281.7	37
37	.220	.288	9.23	.005	.005	−.49	.007	.006	−.14	281.7	38
38	.225	.291	8.86	.005	.003	−1.72	.007	.004	−1.43	283.8	39
39	.230	.295	8.55	.005	.003	−1.45	.007	.005	−1.16	285.1	40
40	.235	.298	8.20	.005	.003	−1.68	.007	.004	−1.41	287.1	41
41	.240	.301	7.95	.005	.004	−1.15	.007	.005	−.86	287.9	42
42	.245	.303	7.50	.005	.002	−2.40	.007	.003	−2.18	292.6	43
43	.250	.307	7.35	.005	.004	−.59	.007	.006	−.30	292.7	44
44	.255	.310	7.01	.005	.003	−1.85	.007	.004	−1.62	295.3	45
45	.260	.314	6.80	.005	.004	−1.06	.007	.005	−.80	296.0	46
46	.265	.317	6.59	.005	.003	−1.04	.007	.005	−.79	296.6	47
47	.270	.319	6.19	.005	.002	−2.31	.007	.003	−2.12	301.1	48
48	.274	.323	6.04	.005	.004	−.73	.007	.006	−.49	301.3	49
49	.279	.325	5.70	.005	.002	−2.02	.007	.003	−1.82	304.6	50
50	.284	.328	5.49	.005	.003	−1.21	.007	.005	−1.00	305.6	51
51	.289	.329	5.00	.005	.001	−3.03	.007	.001	−2.89	314.0	52
52	.293	.332	4.72	.005	.003	−1.70	.007	.004	−1.52	316.3	53
53	.298	.334	4.33	.005	.002	−2.47	.007	.002	−2.33	321.7	54
54	.303	.336	3.99	.005	.002	−2.19	.007	.003	−.2.05	325.9	55
55	.307	.337	3.58	.005	.001	−2.70	.007	.002	−2.59	332.6	56
56	.312	.340	3.37	.005	.003	−1.35	.007	.004	−1.22	334.1	57
57	.316	.342	3.12	.005	.003	−1.60	.007	.004	−1.48	336.3	58
58	.321	.344	2.81	.005	.002	−2.12	.007	.003	−2.02	340.4	59
59	.325	.346	2.46	.004	.002	−2.37	.007	.002	−2.28	345.6	60
60	.330	.348	2.19	.004	.002	−1.81	.007	.003	−1.73	348.6	61
61	.334	.352	2.05	.004	.003	−.98	.007	.005	−.89	349.3	62
62	.338	.354	1.79	.004	.002	−1.77	.007	.004	−1.70	352.2	63
63	.343	.356	1.55	.004	.002	−1.76	.007	.004	−1.69	355.1	64
64	.347	.358	1.26	.004	.002	−2.01	.007	.003	−1.96	358.9	65
65	.351	.361	1.06	.004	.003	−1.44	.007	.004	−1.40	360.9	66
66	.356	.363	.83	.004	.002	−1.70	.007	.004	−1.66	363.7	67
67	.360	.365	.52	.004	.002	−2.24	.007	.003	−2.21	368.6	68
68	.364	.366	.18	.004	.001	−2.50	.007	.002	−2.48	374.7	69
69	.368	.367	−.11	.004	.002	−2.20	.007	.003	−2.20	379.6	70
70	.373	.369	−.44	.004	.001	−2.47	.007	.002	−2.47	385.7	71

$$F(30.5) = 1 - e^{-30.5\,\theta}, \tag{3.8}$$

using Equation 3.4 for the exponential cdf. Our estimate of θ from the 1978 estimation sample equals .006612. Inserting this in Equation 3.8, we get $F(30.5) = .1827$.

The next row, headed cdf, gives the actual proportion of the 1978 validation sample that has returned to prison within the number of months indicated. For example, 806 individuals in the 1978 validation sample had values of TIME of 30 or less. Thus the entry in the row corresponding to 30 months is 806/3,078 = .262; 26.2% of the cohort had returned to prison within 30 (actually 30.5) months. Equivalently stated, the actual 30 month recidivism rate for our 1978 validation sample is 26%.

The next column, headed t, gives the t-statistic used to test the statistical significance of the difference between the predicted and the actual cdf. For a given number of months after release, let p be the actual proportion of individuals who have returned to prison (e.g., .262), and let p^* be the proportion predicted by the model (e.g., .182). Then the test statistic is:

$$(p^* - p)/[p^*(1 - p^*)/n]^{1/2}, \tag{3.9}$$

where n is the number of individuals in the sample (e.g., 3,078). This is equivalent to the statistic given by Schmidt and Witte (1984, p. 114). Under the null hypothesis that the model is correct, the statistic should be distributed as $N(0,1)$ for large n.[3] The value of 11.38, given in the row corresponding to 30 months, exceeds the critical points of $N(0,1)$ for any reasonable level of significance, indicating that the difference between the actual and the predicted cdf is highly significant. This is a reflection of the fact that the exponential distribution is not adequate for our data, as we will discuss later in more detail.

The next three columns of Table 3.1 give essentially the same information as the previous three columns but for the density as opposed to the cdf of the distribution. The column headed Predicted density gives the predicted proportion of the sample that should return to prison during the month in question. For example, again recalling the rule for rounding the data to the nearest whole month, the proportion of the sample which should have TIME = 30 is predicted to be:

$$F(30.5) - F(29.5) = .0055,$$

which is rounded to .005 in Table 3.1. Incidentally, a calculation which is almost equivalent is the density function itself; in this case, $f(30) = .0054$, using Equation 3.3 and a value of .006612 for θ. The column headed Density gives the actual proportion of the sample that returned to prison during each month. For example, for 30 months after release (i.e., TIME

[3] The statistic is therefore not literally a t-statistic. It is, however, equivalent to a t-statistic for large sample sizes. Our sample sizes are indeed large.

= 30), the proportion is 13/3078 = .0042. Finally, the column headed t again gives the t-statistic used to test the statistical significance of the difference between the actual and the predicted density. The statistic is given again by Equation 3.9, except that now p^* is the predicted density and p is the actual density; it is again distributed as $N(0,1)$ for large sample sizes, under the null hypothesis that the model is correct. Therefore, the value of −.91, in the row corresponding to 30 months after release, indicates that the difference between the actual and the predicted density (at time 30) is not statistically significant at usual confidence levels.

The next three columns in Table 3.1 give similar information, but for the hazard rate as opposed to the cdf or density. The column headed Predicted hazard gives the predicted hazard rate for each month after release. For example, the entry in the row corresponding to 30 months after release is calculated as:

$$[F(30.5) - F(29.5)]/[1 - F(29.5)] = .0067,$$

again taking note of the fact that TIME = 30 actually represents recidivism between times 29.5 and 30.5 months. (The calculation of the hazard rate ignoring such considerations would be:

$$f(30)/[1 - F(30)] = .0066,$$

which is quite similar.) The column headed Hazard gives the actual hazard rate for each month after release. For example, for 30 months after release, the actual hazard rate is 13/2285 = .0057, as 13 individuals had TIME = 30 and 2,285 individuals were still at risk at the beginning of month 30. Finally, the column headed t gives the t-statistic used to test the statistical significance of the difference between the predicted and the actual hazard. It is again given by Equation 3.9, with p^* and p now interpreted as the predicted and the actual hazard. The appropriate distribution is again $N(0,1)$ for large sample sizes, under the null hypothesis that the model is correct. Thus the value of −.53, in the row corresponding to 30 months, indicates that the difference between the predicted and the actual hazard (at 30 months after release) is not statistically significant at usual confidence levels.

The last two columns in Table 3.1 give chi-squared statistics (and associated degrees of freedom) that we can use for an overall test of goodness of fit. Since the actual hazard rates for different months are statistically independent, the corresponding t-statistics [actually asymptotic $N(0,1)$ statistics] are also independent across months. If we square these t-statistics and add them up, say over the first m months, we have a statistic whose asymptotic distribution is chi-squared with m degrees of freedom (again, under the null hypothesis that the model is correct). Though this is true for any number of months after return (any value of m), the most interesting value to consider is the full length of the period for which predictions are made. For example, in Table 3.1, the entry in the last row gives a value of 385.7 for the chi-squared statistic with 71 degrees of freedom. This value exceeds the critical points of a chi-squared distribution with 71 degrees of freedom, at any reasonable confidence level, and again indicates that the exponential model is inadequate for our data.

One difficulty that we encounter with some distributions (though not with exponential) is that the predicted hazard rates may be very small, especially long after release, so that the predicted numbers of individuals in some of our "cells" may be quite small. We adopt the standard solution of requiring at least five individuals (predicted) for each cell, which we achieve by combining adjacent months after release as necessary.

We will also make predictions of recidivism using models which include demographic characteristics of individuals as explanatory variables. In this case, the probability distribution of time until recidivism varies over individuals. This affects some of the details of the construction of tables like Table 3.1, though it does not affect their interpretation. For example, consider the problem of predicting the cdf and testing whether the predicted cdf differs significantly from the actual cdf. For a given number of months after release, let R be the actual number of individuals who have returned to prison. (If p is the actual proportion who have returned to prison, as above, and n is the size of the sample, then $R = np$.) Now let p_i^* be the probability implied by the model that individual i should have returned to prison by this time after release. The predicted number of recidivists in the sample of size n is then:

$$\sum_{i=1}^{n} p_i^*, \tag{3.10}$$

and the predicted *proportion* of recidivists is just the result of Equation 3.10 divided by n. The t-statistic used to test the significance of the difference between the predicted and the actual number of recidivists (or equivalently, between the predicted and the actual proportion of recidivists) becomes:

$$\left(\sum_{i=1}^{n} p_i^* - R\right) / \left[\sum_{i=1}^{n} p_i^*(1 - p_i^*)\right]^{1/2}. \tag{3.11}$$

This is exactly the statistic given by Schmidt and Witte (1984, p. 114), which is equivalent to the statistic in Equation 3.9 above if p_i^* is the same for every individual (i.e., if p_i^* does not depend on i). Essentially identical comments apply, of course, to the calculation of the predicted density and hazard rate for the sample, as well as to the calculation of the corresponding test statistics.

For ease of reference, and to provide a preview of our empirical results of the next four chapters, Table 3.2 presents summary measures of the goodness of fit of each of the models we will consider in this book. The name of the model is given as the first entry in each row; for example, the

TABLE 3.2. Summary of predictions.

Model	Individual characteristics?	1978			1980			Using 1978 to predict for 1980	
		ln L	χ^2	$\lvert F-\hat{F}\rvert$	ln L	χ^2	$\lvert F-\hat{F}\rvert$	χ^2	$\lvert F-\hat{F}\rvert$
Nonparametric	N	—	130.3	.012	—	222.2	.028	273.1	.054
Exponential	N	−3,431	385.7	.081	−3,004	428.0	.075	904.2	.128
Weibull	N	−3,405	268.3	.049	−3,000	349.3	.057	613.7	.098
Lognormal	N	−3,370	142.2	.037	−2,969	172.4	.045	350.3	.085
Log-logistic	N	−3,390	209.6	.040	−2,986	269.0	.049	481.5	.087
La Guerre	N	−3,356	118.2	.020	−2,973	172.1	.031	264.6	.059
Split exponential	N	−3,358	115.2	.024	−2,975	174.2	.028	258.1	.057
Split Weibull	N	−3,346	95.9	.017	−2,964	118.5	.032	228.1	.063
Split lognormal	N	−3,342	50.6	.005	−2,955	53.9	.023	126.3	.053
Split log-logistic	N	−3,341	61.0	.011	−2,959	76.4	.024	163.5	.054
Split LaGuerre	N	−3,349	113.8	.021	−2,968	133.0	.034	262.1	.063
Proportional hazards	Y	—	127.1	.012	—	232.4	.034	197.6	.037
Exponential	Y	−3,326	314.1	.066	−2,894	375.8	.069	563.0	.099
Split exponential	Y	−3,285	161.7	.035	−2,882	266.5	.053	258.1	.057
Logit exponential	Y	−3,273	115.2	.025	−2,873	215.5	.042	210.4	.042
Logit/individual exponential	Y	−3,255	120.4	.027	−2,865	181.1	.031	193.8	.037
Lognormal	Y	−3,273	142.5	.034	−2,869	181.9	.051	245.0	.063
Split lognormal	Y	−3,265	110.7	.030	−2,868	173.9	.050	197.0	.057
Logit lognormal	Y	−3,256	50.8	.006	−2,853	57.1	.024	97.6	.042
Logit/individual lognormal	Y	−3,239	51.0	.007	−2,846	62.9	.028	61.8	.032
Logit/individual lognormal (reduced specification)	Y	−3,241	51.6	.013	−2,851	60.0	.027	66.3	.029

results just described for the exponential model are given in the second row of the table. We next indicate whether the model contains (Y) or does not contain (N) individual characteristics as explanatory variables. The models that do not contain explanatory variables are listed first, at the top of the table.

The first three columns of numbers, under the heading "1978," correspond to the case in which the model is estimated using data from the 1978 estimation sample and is used to make predictions for the 1978 validation sample. The first of these columns, labelled "$\ln L$," gives the maximized value of the log likelihood. For example, for the exponential model the maximized value of the log likelihood is – 3,431. The absolute magnitude of this statistic is uninteresting, but a larger value indicates that a model fits the 1978 estimation sample better. However, this statistic is not very useful when comparing models with different numbers of parameters; like the statistic R^2 in a least squares regression, it tends to get larger as the number of parameters increases.

The next column, labelled "χ^2," contains the χ^2 statistic described earlier in this section. For example, for the exponential model the χ^2 statistic equals 385.7, as reported earlier in Table 3.1. A smaller value indicates that the model predicts the recidivism rate in the 1978 validation sample more accurately.

Our final measure of goodness of fit is in the next column, labelled "$|F - \hat{F}|$." It is the maximum difference between the actual and the predicted cumulative distribution function. (In other words, it is the maximum difference between the actual and the predicted recidivism rates.) Except for the fact that our data are censored, this would be the Kolmogorov-Smirnov statistic for goodness of fit. For the exponential model, the statistic equals .081; a glance at Table 3.1 shows that this corresponds to the difference between the actual recidivism rate (cdf) of .258 and the predicted recidivism rate of .177, 29 months after release. A smaller value of this statistic clearly indicates that the model predicts the recidivism rate in the 1978 validation sample more accurately.

The next three columns of numbers, under the heading "1980," correspond to the case in which the model is estimated using data from the 1980 estimation sample and is used to make predictions for the 1980 validation sample. Their interpretation is exactly the same as for the corresponding "1978" results. Finally, the last two columns of numbers, under the heading "Using 1978 to predict for 1980," correspond to the case in which the model is estimated using data from the 1978 estimation sample but is used to make predictions for the 1980 validation sample. Thus the statistics in the last two columns of the table measure the accuracy of predictions across different years of release.

A detailed explanation of the contents of Table 3.2 constitutes the major part of this book. However, to whet the reader's appetite, we note a few salient features of the results displayed there. First, the choice of model makes an enormous difference. Though our best models predict recidivism quite accurately, the majority of the models considered are very inaccurate and potentially misleading. Second, only "split models," of the type introduced by Maltz and McCleary (1977) and discussed in detail in Chapters 5 and 7, perform adequately. Third, when we use data from a release cohort to predict recidivism for individuals in the same release cohort, models with explanatory variables do not predict more accurately than models without explanatory variables. However, explanatory variables are very useful in accounting for differences in recidivism rates across different release cohorts. This is an important finding, because predictions are almost always made using models that have been estimated using data from prior years; a model that cannot predict accurately across different release cohorts is not of much use.

4
Simple Models

Introduction

In this chapter, we will estimate simple models of the length of time until recidivism with data from the 1978 and 1980 estimation samples, and we will see how well these models predict time until recidivism in the corresponding validation samples. The work in this chapter is best seen as a replication and substantial extension of the approach that originated with Stollmack and Harris (1974) and that has been extended by Maltz (1984) and others. This approach seeks to model the timing of recidivism simply by fitting a particular distribution to the data. There is no consideration of explanatory variables, and the goal is just to predict the timing of recidivism for random samples of releasees as accurately as possible. Such predictions can be quite useful; for example, in making projections of future prison populations, they allow one to predict how many releasees will return to prison and when they will do so. However, the models of this chapter cannot predict accurately for non-random samples or make predictions for individuals. Thus their usefulness is somewhat limited.

To be more specific, we will consider nonparametric (model-free) predictions, as well as models based on the exponential, lognormal, log-logistic, Weibull, and LaGuerre distributions. Exponential models have been used widely to analyze time until recidivism; as noted previously, their use dates back to the pioneering work of Stollmack and Harris (1974). Harris and Moitra (1978) used the Weibull distribution to model recidivism. This distribution contains the exponential as a special case, thus providing a more general approach to modeling recidivism than that used by Stollmack and Harris. However, the Weibull distribution still has a monotonic hazard rate and is therefore unlikely to be satisfactory in modeling recidivism. After a considerable search of the relevant statistical literature, we selected the three other distributions that we used (lognormal, log-logistic, and LaGuerre.)[1] We had already used the lognormal distribution to model time until recidivism in a different but similar context (Schmidt & Witte, 1976, 1978, 1980, 1984; Witte & Schmidt, 1977).

Apparently, the latter two distributions had not been used previously to model recidivism. The log-logistic model has been suggested, in the statistical literature on survival times, as an alternative to the lognormal; for example, see Cox and Oates (1984, p. 21). The LaGuerre distribution is a generalization of the exponential that allows a nonmonotonic hazard rate. This distribution can be found in the survival time literature (Cox & Oates, 1984, p. 20), but it is better known in the econometric literature (Schmidt & Mann, 1977; Goldfeld & Quandt, 1981; Kiefer, 1985).

We call the models of this chapter *simple* models because they do not use individual characteristics as explanatory variables and because they are not "split models" in the sense of Maltz and McCleary (1977). We will consider split models in Chapter 5 and models with explanatory variables in Chapters 6 and 7.

Nonparametric Predictions

In this section, we consider a "model" that is not really a model at all in the usual sense of the word. For each of the two validation samples (1978 and 1980), we simply predict that the proportion of recidivists will be the same, in each month, as in the corresponding estimation sample. For example, in the 1978 estimation sample, the proportion of individuals who returned to prison by the end of the 30th month after release is .264 (this is the cumulative distribution function), the proportion of individuals who returned to prison during month 30 is .005 (this is the density), and the proportion of individuals who were still at risk at the beginning of month 30 and who returned to prison during month 30 is .006 (this is the hazard rate). We simply predict these same proportions for the 1978 validation sample.

---

[1] In addition to the distributions that we used in this chapter, we considered and rejected a number of other distributions. The Pareto distribution has a tail that is thicker than the tail of the exponential distribution, and we know from our results (see the section The Exponential Distribution in this chapter) that this is thicker than observed in our data. The density in the tail of the distribution of the timing of recidivism tends to be quite small because most of the individuals who fail tend to do so relatively quickly.

The gamma distribution is often used in survival analyses, but it has two serious defects. First, its hazard rate is monotonic, and our hazard rate is not. Second, its estimation is complicated because evaluation of the distribution function requires evaluation of the incomplete gamma function.

The Gompertz-Makeham distribution is intended for increasing hazard rate applications, and it is clearly inappropriate for recidivism data. Finally, the inverse Gaussian and the generalized *F* distributions are extremely complex.

A good reference for these and other distributions commonly used in survival modeling is Cox and Oates (1984).

This apporach is used extensively and is often referred to as the "life-table" approach because it forms the basis for many actuarial studies. Adler and Kandel (1983) provide an example of a recent use of this approach in criminal justice.

Figure 4.1 illustrates these nonparametric predictions for the 1978 data set. The solid line shows the actual density for the 1978 validation sample. (That is, for any number of months after release, it shows the proportion of the individuals in the validation sample who returned to prison during that month.) The dashed line shows the predicted density for the 1978 validation sample, which is the same as the actual density for the 1978 estimation sample.

Because the estimation and validation samples were defined by a purely random subdivision of the complete data sample, there should be no systematic differences between them. This expectation is borne out in Figure 4.1. There are overpredictions and underpredictions, but there is no apparent systematic pattern to these prediction errors.

Because the differences between the actual and predicted proportions of recidivists are due only to chance, they should be no larger than can

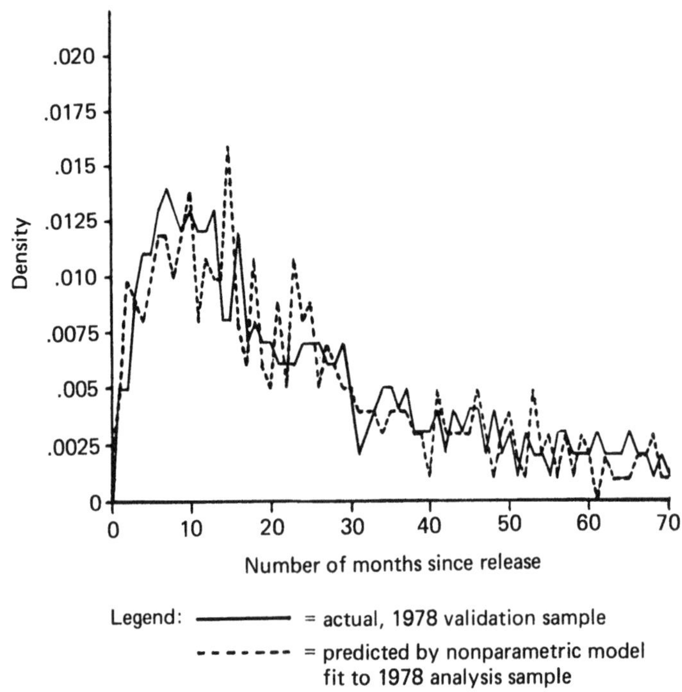

FIGURE 4.1. Predicted versus actual recidivism in the 1978 validation sample: nonparametric model.

reasonably be expected by chance. A statistical test of the significance of such differences is obviously needed. For the parametric models considered in the rest of this chapter, and in Chapters 5 and 7, the t-statistics and chi-squared statistics discussed in Chapter 3 are appropriate for such tests. However, these tests are *not valid* in the present context, even in large samples. The reason is that they treat the predicted proportions as nonrandom (given by the model); they account for the randomness of the actual outcomes but not for the randomness of the predictions. This is not a problem when the predictions come from a statistical model with only a few parameters to estimate, because the variability of the actual proportions swamps the variability (due to parameter estimation) of the predictions. However, it is a problem in the present context. Indeed, because the analysis samples are smaller than the validation samples, the variability of the predicted proportions actually exceeds the variability of the realized proportions. Ignoring this variability will make the differences between the two proportions appear to be much more significant than they really are.

The chi-squared goodness of fit statistic reported for 1978 in Table 3.2 is 130.3. This was calculated as discussed in Chapter 3 and, as just noted, is not a valid test statistic. We report it simply as a numerical measure of goodness of fit, to be used to compare the nonparametric predictions to those based on parametric models. We do so because it is reasonable, in measuring the quality of the predictions, to use the same formula to summarize the nonparametric predictions as that used for predictions based on other models.

Fortunately, an asymptotically valid test is straightforward; we simply use the standard textbook test of the equality of proportions in two populations. When this is done, the chi-squared statistic for 1978 equals 71.5. This does not exceed the critical values of the chi-squared distribution with 61 degrees of freedom, at usual confidence levels, and indicates that the differences between the 1978 validation and estimation samples are no larger than should be expected by chance. Furthermore, the predicted cdf is quite close to the actual cdf, with a maximum difference of only .012. This is about one fourth of the difference that would be required for significance at the 5% level, using the usual Kolmogorov-Smirnov test for equality of two distributions; however, some caution in using this test is necessary due to the censoring of the samples.

As would be expected, the predictions for 1980 are less satisfactory than those for 1978. The maximum difference between the predicted and the actual cdf is .028, which is almost significant at the 10% level using the standard Kolmogorov-Smirnov test (ignoring the censoring). The chi-squared statistic reported in Table 3.2 equals 222.2, which is considerably larger than the corresponding value for 1978. The asymptotically valid chi-squared statistic of 51.3 (with 45 degrees of freedom) is insignificant at usual confidence levels. Nevertheless, there is a noticeable tendency to underpredict the rate of recidivism in the 1980 validation sample. This corresponds to the fact (reported in Chapter 2) that the average value for length of time until return to prison (TIME) is significantly higher in the 1980 validation sample than in the 1980 estimation sample, due simply to bad luck in the subdivision of the 1980 complete data sample. As we will see, our parametric models also predict less well for 1980 than for 1978, because they too tend to underpredict the recidivism rate in the 1980 validation sample.

For both years, the predictions of the density and hazard tend to be less satisfactory than the predictions of the cdf. The problem with the predictions of the density and hazard is that they are too "noisy," in the sense that they simply have too much month-to-month variability. This variability is evident in Figure 4.1. As a specific example, consider the predicted densities for months 10–16, for 1978: .014, .008, .011, .010, .010, .016, and .008. The value of .016 for month 15 is clearly an outlier, representing a (presumably random) "blip" in the experience of the 1978 estimation sample. It is not reasonable to predict such a "blip" for the validation sample. (Indeed, none occurs, and the non-parametric prediction for month 15 is significantly in error.) A similar situation occurs in month 48, where the nonparametric prediction is unreasonably low. Such obvious errors can be avoided by "smoothing" the recidivism rate in the estimation sample before making predictions for the validation sample. This is exactly what is accomplished with a parametric statistical model, as any probability distribution which we assume will have a smooth density and hazard.

The potential problem in using a parametric statistical model, here as elsewhere, is that a model can be (and in practice always is) wrong in the sense that it represents only an approximation to the true distribution being modeled. The predictions from a model can be systematically wrong, and the losses due to this systematic bias have to be weighed against the gains from removing the excess noise of nonparametric predictions. This makes it very important to investigate the adequacy of the models that one assumes. In our case, we will try many different models. Only the best of these will turn out to predict better than we have just done nonparametrically; but these best models do indeed predict *much* better.

One further feature of the empirical distributions of time until recidivism is worth emphasizing at this time. For both years, the hazard rate *rises* for approximately the first six months after release, and then it *falls*. We discussed reasons why this might be the case in Chapters 1 and 2. Such nonmonotonic behavior of the hazard rate is apparently rare in most standard (noncriminological) applications of survival analysis. One can readily find examples of a constant hazard rate (radioactive decay), a rising hazard rate (older light bulbs are more likely to fail), or a decreasing hazard rate (the longer one survives after surgery, the less likely one is to die of complications of the surgery), but a nonmonotonic hazard rate is thought to be unusual. In fact, it is thought to be so unusual that almost none of the standard distributions of survival analysis allow it as a possibility. As we will see, this will lead to some difficulty in finding an adequate distribution to characterize time until recidivism for our data.

The Exponential Distribution

The exponential model has already been covered in some detail in Chapter 3. As noted there, the density and cdf are respectively:

$$\theta e^{-\theta t} \quad \text{and} \quad 1 - e^{-\theta t}.$$

We require $\theta > 0$. The mean of the distribution is $1/\theta$, and the variance is $1/\theta^2$. The hazard rate is a constant, θ; in fact, the exponential distribution is the only distribution with a constant hazard rate.

The standard example of a phenomenon that follows the exponential distribution is the time until a radioactive particle decays. The probability that the particle will decay in the next unit of time is independent of its age, so the hazard rate is constant.

Our data do not display a constant hazard rate, and we should not expect an exponential model to fit them well. Nevertheless, we will consider this model because it is a common one, with some precedent in criminology (e.g., Stollmack & Harris, 1974), and also because it is a good example of how misleading an inadequate model can be.

The formulae for the likelihood function and the maximum likelihood estimate of θ are given in Chapter 3, Equations 3.5 and 3.7. Our estimates of θ, the hazard rate, are .006612 and .009382 for 1978 and 1980, respectively. The estimated failure rate is higher in the 1980 data, in this model as in all others that we fit. The mean time until recidivism is estimated to be 1/.006612 = 151.2 months for 1978 and 1/.009382 = 104.8 months for 1980. These numbers appear quite high until it is remembered that the time until recidivism has a highly skewed distribution. The median time until recidivism would be considerably below the mean and, in this context, is probably a better measure of central tendency. We also note for future reference that the likelihood values achieved[2] are −3,430.8 for 1978 and −3,004.5 for 1980; these are recorded in Table 3.2.

Table 3.1 (in the previous chapter) gives the results of using our exponential model, estimated on the 1978 estimation sample, to make predictions for the 1978 validation sample. We do not display the corresponding 1980 results, but they are quite similar. The results are rather poor, reflecting the fact that the exponential distribution does not fit the data well. The maximum difference between the predicted and the actual cdf is

---

[2] That is, the *maximized* value of the likelihood.

.081 for 1978 and .075 for 1980; each is much larger than the corresponding value for our nonparametric predictions. The chi-squared values are also much larger; 385.7 for 1978 and 428.0 for 1980. (Both sets of goodness of fit statistics are recorded in Table 3.2.) Many of the differences between the predicted and the actual proportions (in terms of cdf, density, or hazard) of recidivists are statistically significant. In terms of density or hazard, the exponential model predicts too many recidivists immediately after release (for the first month or two) and for periods long after release (past 25 to 30 months, say), but it predicts too few recidivists during the intermediate period. In terms of cdf, the exponential model underpredicts the proportion of recidivists for all periods except the first few and (for 1978) the last few.

The poor performance of the model using the exponential distribution is exactly as expected. Our data have a hazard rate that first rises and then falls, whereas the exponential distribution assumes a constant hazard. Distributions with a nonconstant hazard generally will be expected to give a better fit to our data.

The Lognormal Model

A random variable has a lognormal distribution if its logarithm has a normal distribution. Thus, in this section, we assume that the logarithm of time until recidivism is normally distributed, with mean μ and variance σ^2. The density of the time until recidivism is therefore:

$$f(t) = \exp[-(1/2\sigma^2)(\ln t - \mu)^2]/(t\sigma\sqrt{2\pi}), \tag{4.1}$$

and the cdf is:

$$F(t) = \Phi[(\ln t - \mu)/\sigma], \tag{4.2}$$

where Φ is the standard normal cdf. The likelihood function is then given by Equation 3.2; see also Schmidt and Witte (1984, p. 91). There is no explicit formula for the maximum likelihood estimates of μ and σ^2; they must be found by a numerical maximization of the likelihood. The lognormal model has been used previously by Amemiya and Boskin (1974), Schmidt and Witte (1976, 1978, 1979, 1980, 1984), and Witte and Schmidt (1977).

The lognormal distribution has a hazard rate that first rises and then falls. This is the same pattern found in our data, so there is some reason to hope that the lognormal distribution may fit adequately. Indeed, this is one of the reasons we adopted this model in our early work.

The maximum likelihood estimates of μ and σ^2 are, respectively, 4.9168 and 3.9708 for 1978 and 4.4974 and 3.2234 for 1980. These imply strikingly large mean values of time until recidivism: 994 months for 1978 and 449 months for 1980. (The median values, which we found to be a more meaningful measure of central tendency, are however a bit more reasonable, namely 137 months and 90 months.) The likelihood values achieved are −3,369.7 and −2,969.0, as reported in Table 3.2, which are noticeably larger (less negative) than for the exponential model. These values provide convincing evidence that the lognormal model fits our data better than the exponential.

Our predictions for the 1978 and 1980 validation samples using the estimated lognormal models are much better than for the exponential model, as expected. The maximum differences between the predicted and actual cdf's are .037 for 1978 and .045 for 1980 (see Table 3.2), and these are much smaller than the corresponding values for the exponential case, though still larger than for the non-parametric predictions. The overall chi-squared statistics of 142.2 and 172.4 are also much smaller than the values for the exponential case, though again they are larger than the values for the nonparametric predictions.

Although the lognormal model fits better than the exponential model, it is still not very good. In terms of density or hazard, it exhibits (to a lesser degree) the same flaw as the exponential model: it overpredicts recidivism in the early months after release and in the tail, and it underpredicts recidivism for the period in between. This pattern can be seen clearly in Figure 4.2, in which the solid line represents the actual density of time until recidivism in the 1978 validation sample, and the dotted line represents the density predicted by the lognormal model fit to the 1978 estimation sample. The prediction errors are not always significantly different from zero, but they are systematic and noticeable. In terms of cdf, the lognormal model underpredicts recidivism for all except the first 6 months or so. Many of these prediction errors are very significantly different from zero. These results convinced us that we needed to search for alternative statistical models to model the timing of recidivism properly.

Overall, the performance of the lognormal model is disappointing. Qualitatively, its hazard has the right features, in that it rises and then falls; however, it does not fall fast enough to fit our data adequately. Indeed, as we will see, this turns out to be a problem with all of the simple models that we consider.

The Log-Logistic Model

The log-logistic distribution is related to the logistic distribution in the same way that the lognormal distribution is related to the normal. A random variable has a log-logistic distribution if its logarithm has a logistic distribution. The logistic distribution is quite similar to the normal, except in the tails, so we should expect the log-logistic distribution to be fairly similar to the lognormal. As far as we are aware, the log-logistic distribution has not been used previously to model the timing of recidivism.

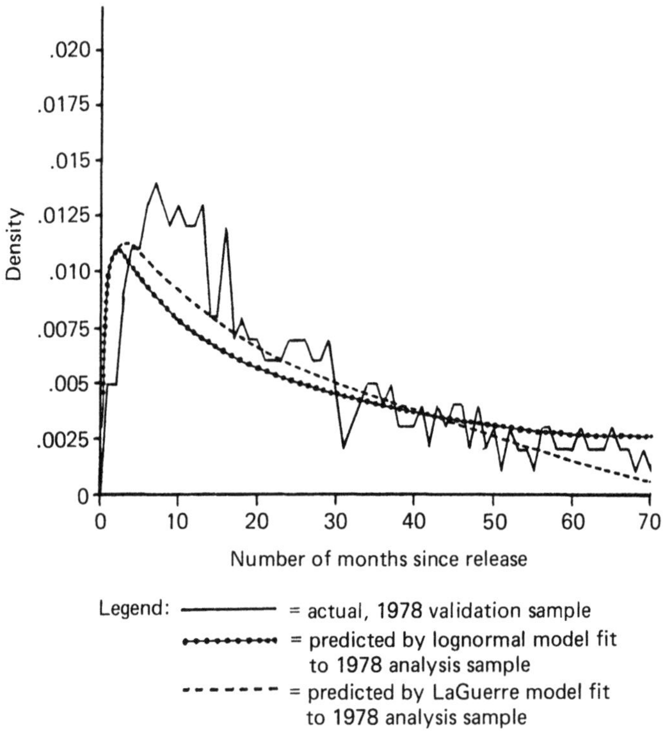

FIGURE 4.2. Predicted versus actual recidivism in the 1978 validation sample: lognormal and LaGuerre models.

The log-logistic distribution depends on two parameters, α and k, both of which must be positive. Its density, cdf, and hazard are given by:

$$f(t) = k\alpha^k t^{k-1}/[1 + (\alpha t)^k]^2, \tag{4.3}$$

$$1 - F(t) = 1/[1 + (\alpha t)^k], \tag{4.4}$$

and

$$h(t) = k\alpha^k t^{k-1}/[1 + (\alpha t)^k] \tag{4.5}$$

(see e.g., Cox & Oates, 1984, p. 21). The hazard decreases monotonically if $k < 1$ and has a single maximum if $k > 1$. Therefore, the log-logistic hazard can take on the same qualitative features (first increasing and then decreasing) as the hazard in our data has.

The maximum likelihood estimates of α and k are .007858 and .87494 for 1978 and .01189 and .9783 for 1980. It is interesting that for each year the estimated value for k implies a monotonically decreasing hazard. Our data do not have a monotonically decreasing hazard, so we might have expected to find a value of k greater than one, which would imply a hazard that rose and then fell. This did not occur, and the reasonable explanation is that with $k > 1$ the falling portion of the hazard would not fall fast enough to provide a good fit to the tail of our data. As we have noted, an important aspect of our data is that the hazard rate falls very rapidly once it begins to fall.

The likelihood values achieved, as reported in Table 3.2, are −3,390.1 and −2,986.0, indicating a worse fit than with the lognormal model (for each year). The log-logistic predictions for the 1978 and 1980 validation samples are also worse than for the lognormal model, as is clear from the goodness of fit statistics reported in Table 3.2. The maximum differences between the predicted and the actual cdf are .040 and .049, which are slightly larger than the corresponding values for the lognormal model. The overall chi-squared statistics are 209.6 and 269.0, which are considerably larger than the lognormal values.

The problem with the fit of the log-logistic distribution to our data is essentially the same as the problem with the exponential and lognormal distributions. It overpredicts the hazard and density at the very first and in the tail, and it underpredicts in between. Correspondingly, it underpredicts the cdf, except for the first few months. These problems with the log-logistic distribution are less severe than with the exponential but more severe than with the lognormal.

The Weibull Model

The Weibull distribution is a well-known generalization of the exponential distribution, and it is used widely in survival analysis. See Harris and Moitra (1978) for an example of its use in a criminal justice application. A random variable t has a Weibull distribution if t^k has an exponential distribution, for some k greater than zero. The Weibull distribution has density, cdf, and hazard given by:

$$f(t) = k\theta^k \, t^{k-1} \, e^{-(\theta t)^k}, \tag{4.6}$$

$$F(t) = 1 - e^{-(\theta t)^k}, \tag{4.7}$$

and

$$h(t) = k\theta^k t^{k-1}. \tag{4.8}$$

The hazard is monotonically decreasing if $k < 1$ and monotonically increasing if $k > 1$. If $k = 1$, we are back to the exponential distribution, and the hazard is constant.

The maximum likelihood estimates of θ and k are .005090 and .7672 for 1978 and .008171 and .8633 for 1980. These values imply a falling hazard rate, as expected. Because k does not equal one, our results do not reduce to the exponential. This is further evidence that the exponential distribution is not appropriate for our data.

The likelihood values achieved were −3,405.5 for 1978 and −2,999.6 for 1980, as reported in Table 3.2. This indicates a better fit than the exponential distribution,[3] but a worse fit than the lognormal or log-logistic distributions. This is to be expected since the Weibull imposes a monotonic hazard rate.

The predictions for the 1978 and 1980 validation samples tell more or less the same story. The maximum differences between the predicted and the actual cdf are .049 and .057, while the overall chi-squared statistics are 268.3 and 349.3. By either measure the fit is better than for the exponential distribution, but worse than for the lognormal or log-logistic distributions. The basic problem with the Weibull distribution's fit is exactly as for the other distributions considered so far. It overpredicts hazard and density at first and in the tail, but underpredicts in between; it underpredicts the cdf, except for the first few months. The goodness of fit statistics reported in Table 3.2 indicate that these problems are fairly severe for the Weibull distribution; less serve than for the exponential, and more severe than for the lognormal or log-logistic distributions.

The LaGuerre Model

The last simple model that we will consider is a rather uncommon one that we will refer to as the LaGuerre model. This is not an entirely standard nomenclature and, indeed, there does not seem to be one. The LaGuerre distribution can be found in Cox and Oates (1984, p. 20), Kiefer (1985), and Goldfeld and Quandt (1981). Its density is the product of an exponential function and a polynomial, which is known as a LaGuerre polynomial in the mathematical literature. The exponential guarantees that the density approaches zero in the tail, while the the polynomial allows some flexibility in the distribution, especially for small values of t. How much flexibility is allowed naturally depends on the degree of the polynomial.

One reason why the LaGuerre distribution may be attractive is that, for a sufficiently high degree of its polynomial, it can approximate *any* survival time distribution arbitrarily well. Such approximation results are given by Schmidt and Mann (1977), who relied on a theorem developed by Stone (1962), and also given by Lutkepohl (1980). On the other hand, one reason why the LaGuerre distribution may be unattractive is that it is sometimes *too* flexible; there is no simple way to ensure that the density will be nonnegative for all values of t. In maximizing the likelihood function, one simply must rule out parameter values that do not lead to a

[3] Since the Weibull distribution contains the exponential distribution as a special case, it cannot fit the data worse than the exponential does.

(globally) nonnegative density, and this is a potentially complicated set of restrictions.

We will use a second-degree LaGuerre distribution. This allows a single "turning point," which is what we observe in our data. Its density, cdf, and hazard are given by:

$$f(t) = \alpha(1 + \delta_1 \alpha t + \delta_2 \alpha^2 t^2)e^{-\alpha t}/d, \tag{4.9}$$

$$F(t) = 1 - e^{-\alpha t} - \alpha t(\delta_1 + 2\delta_2)\, e^{-\alpha t}/d - \alpha^2 t^2 \delta_2 e^{-\alpha t}/d, \tag{4.10}$$

and

$$h(t) = \alpha(1 + \delta_1 \alpha t + \delta_2 \alpha^2 t^2)/[d + \alpha t(\delta_1 + 2\delta_2) + \alpha^2 t^2 \delta_2], \tag{4.11}$$

where $d = 1 + \delta_1 + 2\delta_2$. We require $\alpha > 0$. As discussed earlier, we also require the density to be nonnegative for all t, which implies some restrictions on δ_1 and δ_2. These restrictions are imposed in the numerical maximization of the likelihood function.

The maximum likelihood estimates of α, δ_1 and δ_2 were .008463, −1.869, and .7888 for 1978, and .005077, −3.429, and 1.4013 for 1980. The likelihood values achieved were −3,355.8 and −2,973.2, respectively. For 1978, this is the highest likelihood value yet achieved (see the first six rows of Table 3.2), indicating that the LaGuerre model provides the best fit so far to the 1978 estimation sample. For 1980, on the other hand, the likelihood value is slightly lower than that achieved by the lognormal model.

The LaGuerre model's predictions for the 1978 and 1980 validation samples are displayed in Tables 4.1 and 4.2; the predicted density for 1978 is also displayed as the dashed line in Figure 4.2. For each year, the LaGuerre model provides better predictions of the recidivism rate in the validation sample than any of the other parametric models yet considered. The maximum differences between the predicted and the actual cdf are .020 for 1978 and .031 for 1980. These are noticeably smaller than the corresponding values for our other distributions (though they are larger than the values for the nonparametric predictions), as can be seen in Table 3.2. The overall chi-squared statistics are 118.2 for 1978 and 172.1 for 1980, and these are smaller than the overall chi-squared statistics for any of our other distributions or for the nonparametric predictions. As can be seen in Figure 4.2 or in Tables 4.1 and 4.2, the LaGuerre model overpredicts the rate of recidivism for the first few months after release, as did all of our other parametric models. It then underpredicts the rate of recidivism for the next year or so; all of the other models also did this, but they continued to underpredict for a longer time than the LaGuerre model. Unlike our other models, the LaGuerre model fits the tail of the distribution (20 months or more after release, say) reasonably well. There is some tendency to overpredict recidivism in the tail of the 1980 distribution,

TABLE 4.1. Predicted versus actual recidivism rates for 1978 validation sample using LaGuerre model fit to 1978 analysis sample.

N	Predicted cdf	cdf	t	Predicted density	Density	t	Predicted hazard	Hazard	t	χ^2	df
0	.006	.000	−4.29	.006	000	−4.29	.006	.000	−4.29	18.4	1
1	.018	.005	−5.23	.012	.005	−3.34	.012	.005	−3.36	29.7	2
2	.029	.010	−6.36	.011	.005	−3.57	.012	.005	−3.62	42.8	3
3	.040	.019	−5.91	.011	.009	−.89	.011	.010	−.99	43.8	4
4	.051	.031	−5.14	.011	.011	.29	.011	.012	.16	43.8	5
5	.061	.042	−4.51	.011	.011	.44	.011	.012	.32	43.9	6
6	.072	.055	−3.62	.010	.013	1.48	.011	.014	1.35	45.8	7
7	.082	.069	−2.61	.010	.014	2.19	.011	.015	2.07	50.0	8
8	.092	.082	−1.80	.010	.013	1.99	.011	.014	1.90	53.6	9
9	.101	.094	−1.33	.010	.012	1.23	.011	.013	1.17	55.0	10
10	.110	.107	−.68	.009	.013	1.95	.010	.014	1.90	58.6	11
11	.119	.119	−.15	.009	.012	1.73	.010	.013	1.71	61.5	12
12	.128	.131	.44	.009	.012	2.09	.010	.014	2.08	65.9	13
13	.137	.144	−1.08	.009	.013	2.45	.010	.015	2.47	71.9	14
14	.145	.151	.96	.008	.008	−.35	.010	.009	−.31	72.0	15
15	.153	.160	.94	.008	.008	−.02	.010	.010	.01	72.0	16
16	.161	.171	1.48	.008	.012	2.35	.009	.014	2.39	77.8	17
17	.169	.178	1.37	.008	.007	−.37	.009	.009	−.31	77.9	18
18	.177	.186	1.39	.008	.008	.18	.009	.009	.23	77.9	19
19	.184	.193	1.34	.007	.007	−.11	.009	.009	−.06	77.9	20
20	.191	.200	1.28	.007	.007	−.20	.009	.008	−.14	77.9	21
21	.198	.206	1.11	.007	.006	−.72	.009	.007	−.67	78.4	22
22	.205	.212	1.02	.007	.006	−.38	.008	.008	−.34	78.5	23
23	.211	.218	.87	.007	.006	−.70	.008	.007	−.67	79.0	24

24	.218	.224	.92	.006	.007	.32	.008	.009	.36	79.1	25
25	.224	.232	1.04	.006	.007	.68	.008	.009	.72	79.6	26
26	.230	.239	1.18	.006	.007	.82	.008	.009	.87	80.4	27
27	.236	.245	1.21	.006	.006	.25	.008	.008	.30	80.4	28
28	.241	.251	1.23	.006	.006	.13	.007	.008	.19	80.5	29
29	.247	.258	1.39	.006	.007	.99	.007	.009	1.05	81.6	30
30	.252	.262	1.24	.005	.004	−.85	.007	.006	−.80	82.2	31
31	.257	.264	.86	.005	.002	−2.25	.007	.003	−2.21	87.1	32
32	.262	.267	.55	.005	.003	−1.90	.007	.004	−1.88	90.6	33
33	.267	.271	.46	.005	.004	−.52	.007	.006	−.50	90.9	34
34	.272	.276	.44	.005	.005	−.14	.006	.006	−.12	90.9	35
35	.277	.280	.43	.005	.005	−.03	.006	.006	−.01	90.9	36
36	.281	.284	.36	.004	.004	−.45	.006	.005	−.43	91.1	37
37	.285	.288	.39	.004	.005	.21	.006	.006	.23	91.1	38
38	.289	.291	.24	.004	.003	−1.07	.006	.004	−1.05	92.2	39
39	.293	.295	.14	.004	.003	−.68	.006	.005	−.67	92.7	40
40	.297	.298	.03	.004	.003	−.87	.006	.004	−.86	93.4	41
41	.301	.301	.00	.004	.004	−.18	.005	.005	−.18	93.5	42
42	.305	.303	−.20	.004	.002	−1.56	.005	.003	−1.56	95.9	43
43	.308	.307	−.12	.004	.004	.66	.005	.006	.65	96.3	44
44	.312	.310	−.21	.003	.003	−.77	.005	.004	−.77	96.9	45
45	.315	.314	−.18	.003	.004	.28	.005	.005	.27	97.0	46
46	.318	.317	−.13	.003	.004	.40	.005	.005	.39	97.1	47
47	.321	.319	−.26	.003	.002	−1.12	.004	.003	−1.12	98.4	48

TABLE 4.1. *Continued.*

N	Predicted cdf	cdf	t	Predicted density	Density	t	Predicted hazard	Hazard	t	χ^2	df
48	.324	.323	−.15	.003	.004	.97	.004	.006	.96	99.3	49
49	.327	.325	−.22	.003	.002	−.59	.004	.003	−.60	99.7	50
50	.330	.328	−.16	.003	.003	.54	.004	.005	.53	100.0	51
51	.332	.329	−.35	.003	.001	−1.80	.004	.001	−1.81	103.2	52
52	.335	.332	−.34	.003	.003	.06	.004	.004	.05	103.2	53
53	.337	.334	−.44	.003	.002	−.92	.004	.002	−.93	104.1	54
54	.340	.336	−.49	.002	.002	−.46	.004	.003	−.47	104.3	55
55	.342	.337	−.60	.002	.001	−1.12	.003	.002	−1.13	105.6	56
56	.344	.340	−.51	.002	.003	.90	.003	.004	.88	106.4	57
57	.346	.342	−.45	.002	.003	.63	.003	.004	.61	106.8	58
58	.348	.344	−.45	.002	.002	−.06	.003	.003	−.07	106.8	59
59	.350	.346	−.48	.002	.002	−.36	.003	.002	−.38	106.9	60
60	.352	.348	−.43	.002	.002	.58	.003	.003	.56	107.2	61
61	.354	.352	−.26	.002	.003	1.99	.003	.005	1.97	111.1	62
62	.355	.354	−.19	.002	.002	.82	.003	.004	.81	111.8	63
63	.357	.356	−.11	.002	.002	.94	.002	.004	.94	—	—
64	.359	.358	−.06	.002	.002	.61	.002	.003	.60	113.0	64
65	.360	.361	.07	.001	.003	1.67	.002	.004	1.67	—	—
66	.361	.363	.18	.001	.002	1.33	.002	.004	1.34	117.5	65
67	.363	.365	.21	.001	.002	.48	.002	.003	.48	—	—
68	.364	.366	.22	.001	.001	.08	.002	.002	.09	117.6	66
69	.365	.367	.27	.001	.002	.71	.002	.003	.72	—	—
70	.366	.369	.29	.001	.001	.30	.002	.002	.30	118.2	67

TABLE 4.2. Predicted versus actual recidivism rates for 1980 validation sample using LaGuerre model fit to 1980 analysis sample.

N	Predicted cdf	cdf	t	Predicted density	Density	t	Predicted hazard	Hazard	t	χ^2	df
0	.007	.001	−4.30	.007	.001	−4.30	.001	.001	−4.30	18.5	1
1	.020	.005	−7.21	.013	.003	−5.75	.013	.003	−5.78	51.8	2
2	.033	.014	−6.93	.013	.010	−2.01	.013	.010	−2.11	56.3	3
3	.046	.030	−5.02	.013	.016	1.68	.013	.016	1.52	58.6	4
4	.058	.046	−3.34	.012	.016	2.43	.013	.017	2.28	63.8	5
5	.070	.064	−1.63	.012	.018	3.32	.013	.019	3.21	74.2	6
6	.082	.079	−.68	.012	.015	2.13	.013	.016	2.07	78.4	7
7	.094	.094	.00	.012	.014	1.76	.013	.016	1.73	81.4	8
8	.105	.111	1.32	.011	.017	3.83	.012	.019	3.83	96.1	9
9	.116	.126	2.11	.011	.015	2.59	.012	.017	2.64	103.1	10
10	127	.141	2.94	.011	.015	2.94	.012	.018	3.04	112.3	11
11	.137	.157	3.77	.010	.015	3.15	.012	.018	3.29	123.2	12
12	.147	.171	4.44	.010	.014	2.76	.012	.017	2.94	131.9	13
13	.157	.183	4.59	.010	.011	.97	.012	.014	1.17	133.2	14
14	.167	.194	4.74	.010	.011	1.00	.011	.014	1.21	134.7	15
15	.176	.205	4.98	.009	.011	1.34	.011	.014	1.57	137.2	16
16	.185	.214	4.86	.009	.009	−.07	.011	.011	.16	137.2	17
17	.194	.224	4.92	.009	.010	.59	.011	.012	.83	137.9	18
18	.203	.234	5.01	.009	.010	.77	.011	.013	1.02	138.9	19
19	.211	.240	4.59	.008	.006	−1.54	.011	.008	−1.34	140.7	20
20	.220	.249	4.71	.008	.009	.81	.010	.012	1.04	141.8	21
21	.228	.257	4.68	.008	.008	.13	.010	.011	.37	141.9	22
22	.235	.262	4.11	.008	.004	−2.48	.010	.006	−2.30	147.2	23
23	.243	.269	3.99	.007	.007	−.39	.010	.009	−.20	147.3	24
24	.250	.274	3.66	.007	.005	−1.48	.010	.007	−1.31	149.0	25
25	.257	.282	3.68	.007	.007	.31	.009	.010	.50	149.2	26
26	.264	.287	3.50	.007	.006	−.80	.009	.008	−.63	149.6	27
27	.270	.294	3.46	.007	.007	−.07	.009	.009	.10	149.6	28
28	.277	.298	3.12	.006	.004	−1.81	.009	.006	−1.67	152.4	29

TABLE 4.2. *Continued.*

N	Predicted cdf	cdf	t	Predicted density	Density	t	Predicted hazard	Hazard	t	χ^2	df
29	.283	.303	2.87	.006	.005	−1.28	.009	.007	−1.14	153.7	30
30	.289	.307	2.56	.006	.004	−1.71	.008	.006	−1.60	156.3	31
31	.295	.311	2.36	.006	.004	−1.16	.008	.006	−1.05	157.4	32
32	.300	.318	2.51	.006	.007	1.05	.008	.010	1.18	158.8	33
33	.306	.322	2.34	.005	.004	−1.05	.008	.006	−.94	159.7	34
34	.311	.327	2.32	.005	.005	−.03	.007	.008	.08	159.7	35
35	.316	.334	2.53	.005	.007	1.45	.007	.010	1.58	162.2	36
36	.320	.338	2.47	.005	.004	−.33	.007	.007	−.21	162.2	37
37	.325	.340	2.15	.005	.002	2.18	.007	.004	−2.10	166.6	38
38	.329	.344	1.98	.004	.003	−1.12	.006	.005	−1.04	167.7	39
39	.334	.348	1.94	.004	.004	−.25	.006	.006	−.16	167.7	40
40	.338	.351	1.86	.004	.003	−.55	.006	.005	−.47	167.9	41
41	.341	.354	1.78	.004	.003	−.62	.006	.005	−.54	168.2	42
42	.345	.357	1.62	.004	.003	−1.20	.006	.004	−1.13	169.5	43
43	.349	.360	1.62	.003	.003	.01	.005	.005	.08	169.5	44
44	.352	.362	1.45	.003	.002	−1.39	.005	.003	−1.34	171.3	45
45	.355	.365	1.33	.003	.002	−.95	.005	.004	−.90	172.1	46
46	.358	.368	1.30	.003	.003	−.22	.005	.004	−.17	172.1	47

though less so than with other models, and there is no noticeable tendency to do so for 1978. Thus, the main improvement in prediction comes in the tail of the distribution, and it occurs because the flexibility of the LaGuerre distribution allows the hazard to fall faster than is possible in the other distributions we considered. This is an important feature for a survival model of recidivism.

Conclusions

Using data from the 1978 and 1980 estimation samples, we have estimated a variety of models and have used them to make predictions of the rate of recidivism in the 1978 and 1980 validation samples. Specifically, we have considered a nonparametric "model," and we have used parametric models based on the exponential, Weibull, lognormal, log-logistic, and LaGuerre distributions.

Our nonparametric "model" simply predicts, for each validation sample, the same distribution of time until recidivism as that found in the corresponding estimation sample. These predictions exhibit no systematic bias, but they are excessively variable. We can hope to improve on them by "smoothing" the density (or hazard) to reduce this month to month variability. Our parametric models are intended to accomplish this smoothing.

The most successful of our parametric models, in terms of goodness of fit to the estimation samples and accuracy of predictions for the validation samples, is the LaGuerre model. However, it is not entirely adequate because it exhibits a clear tendency to overpredict recidivism for the first few months after release and then underpredict recidivism for the next year or so. (All of our other parametric distributions have these same faults; in addition, they tend to overpredict recidivism in the tail of the distribution, which the LaGuerre does not.) Overall, the quality of the predictions from the LaGuerre model is comparable to the quality of the nonparametric predictions. Thus, if one is going to predict recidivism using a simple model of the type used in this chapter, a simple life-table approach may be better than a parametric model. We have not yet succeeded in finding a model which is sufficiently accurate to outpredict the nonparametric "model." It is interesting that this is the case, after trying five different distributions. In the next chapter, we will be more successful as we consider models that allow for the possibility that not all individuals ultimately return to prison.

5
Split Population Models

Introduction

The "simple" parametric models considered in the last chapter have all assumed some form of the cumulative distribution function $F(t)$ for the time until recidivism. Any such cumulative distribution function approaches one as t becomes sufficiently large. In the present context, this implies that every individual would eventually return to prison, and this implicit assumption can be argued to be unreasonable.

In this chapter, we will consider "split population models," as defined by Maltz and McCleary (1977), in which the probability of eventual recidivism is an additional parameter to be estimated and may be less than one. (We will also refer to these models simply as "split models," and the parameter that represents the probability of eventual recidivism will be called the "splitting parameter." In terms of the career criminal paradigm, the termination rate is one minus the value of this parameter.) A distribution of failure times is also specified as before, but this is understood to apply only to those individuals who will fail eventually. Just as the previous chapter could be considered a substantial extension of the work of Stollmack and Harris (1974), this chapter can be considered a substantial extension of the work of Maltz and his colleagues.

Using the notation of Schmidt and Witte (1984, section 6.4), we can express a split model as follows. First, let F be an *unobservable* variable indicating whether an individual would or would not eventually fail. Specifically, let F equal one for individuals who would eventually fail and zero for individuals who would never fail. Then we assume:

$$P(F = 1) = \delta, \ P(F = 0) = 1 - \delta. \tag{5.1}$$

The parameter δ is, of course, the eventual recidivism rate, and $1 - \delta$ is the rate of termination. Second, we assume some cumulative distribution function $G(t|F = 1)$ for the individuals who would ultimately fail, and we let $g(t|F = 1)$ be the corresponding density. We can assume any type of distribution that seems reasonable; in this chapter, we will consider the same distributions that were used in the last chapter (exponential, lognormal, log-logistic, Weibull, and LaGuerre). We note explicitly that such a distribution is defined *conditional* on $F = 1$, and it is irrelevant for individuals for whom $F = 0$—that is, for those individuals who would never return to prison.

Now let T be the length of the follow-up period, and let R be the observable dummy variable indicating whether or not the individual has returned to prison by the end of the follow-up period. We wish to construct a likelihood function for the sample. For the recidivists in the sample, we observe $R = 1$ and the failure time t, and of course we know that $F = 1$. The appropriate density to enter into the likelihood function is therefore:

$$P(F = 1)\ g(t|F = 1) = \delta\ g(t|F = 1). \tag{5.2}$$

(For example, in the exponential case Equation 5.2 equals $\delta\theta e^{-\theta t}$.) On the other hand, for the nonrecidivists in the sample, we observe only $R = 0$, and the probability of this event is:

$$\begin{aligned} P(R = 0) &= P(F = 0) + P(F = 1)\ P(t > T|F = 1) \\ &= 1 - \delta + \delta\,[1 - G(T|F = 1)]. \end{aligned} \tag{5.3}$$

(For example, in Equation 5.3 is $1 - \delta + \delta e^{-\delta t}$.) The first term in this equation reflects the fact that some people will never fail, whereas the second reflects the fact that some people will fail after we cease to observe their activities.

The likelihood is then made up of terms like Equation 5.2 for recidivists and Equation 5.3 for nonrecidivists (individuals who have not returned to prison by the end of the follow-up period). Explicitly, with individuals indexed by $i = 1, \ldots, N$, the likelihood function becomes:

$$\begin{aligned} \ln L = \sum_{i=1}^{N} \{R_i\ [\ln \delta + \ln g(t_i|F_i = 1)] \\ + (1 - R_i) \ln [1 - \delta + \delta\ (1 - G(T_i|F_i = 1))]\} \end{aligned} \tag{5.4}$$

The calculation of the maximum likelihood estimates of the parameters (δ and whatever parameters are in the distribution function G) will generally require a numerical maximization of this likelihood function.

Split models were introduced to the criminological literature by Maltz and McCleary (1977), who considered the exponential case; previous treatments in the statistical literature date back at least to Anscombe (1961). In our opinion, split models are potentially useful whether or not one is willing to accept as meaningful the probability that an individual will "eventually fail." Rather, their potential usefulness stems from the fact that they allow for *heterogeneity* of individuals. Models that treat all individuals as identical, such as those used in the previous chapter, are very likely to overpredict long-term recidivism rates. For example, for the 1980 release cohort, the failure rates 25 years after release which are implied by our models of Chapter 4 are as follows: exponential, .94; lognormal, .78; log-logistic, .78; Weibull, .89; and LaGuerre, .52. All of these except the last seem unreasonably high. By comparison, the split models of this chapter will imply 25-year failure rates on the order of .50.[1]

There is some limited information available that allows one to estimate the eventual rate of recidivism for a release cohort. The ideal of way of obtaining this information would be to follow a cohort from release until death and observe their criminal activity during this period. However, there has been no such study. The longest follow-up of which we are aware is the 30-year follow-up conducted by McCord (1978) in connection with the Cambridge–Sommerville youth study. This study, which began in 1939 when the boys in the sample were approximately 10 years old, involved a program that provided 5 years of counseling. McCord found an official conviction rate of 36% for serious offenses at the end of 30 years. This rate should be considerably below the "eventual" recidivism rate for our sample, as we are dealing with prison releasees rather than youths from a working class neighborhood.

In what is perhaps the most useful study for our purposes, Kitchener, Schmidt, and Glaser (1977) followed for 18 years a sample of individuals who were released from the federal prison system in 1956. Recidivism was defined as return to prison for a parole violation, a felony, or a felony-like offense. They report recidivism rates of 15% for one year after release, 51% for 5 years after release, 59% for 10 years after release, and 63% for 18 years after release. These recidivism rates are not completely comparable to our own because they deal with a different population (federal versus state releasees), a different failure criterion, and a different time period (1956 versus 1978 and 1980). The one-year recidivism rate of Kitchener et al. is quite similar to our own, but their 5 year failure rate is approximately 15% higher than ours. What is most interesting, however, is that the growth of the recidivism rate in their study declines very markedly 3 years after release and is very low for periods longer than 10 years after release. Indeed, the probability of failure for those who had survived 17 years was less than 1% during the 18th year after release. See Hoffman and Stone-Meierhoefer (1979, p. 197) for a discussion of this point.

Hoffman and Stone-Meierhoefer (1979) follow a more recent (1970) cohort of federal releasees for 6 years. They report that 62.5% of their releasees had been arrested, 34% had returned to prison for a sentence of 60 days or more, and 28% had returned to prison for a sentence of 1 year or more.

What do these results tell us about possible values for the eventual recidivism rate (our δ)? This rate is almost certainly greater than the 36%

[1] Our best-fitting model of this chapter, the split lognormal model, implies a 25-year failure rate of .48, for example.

reported by McCord in 1978 (indeed, we observe a recidivism rate of approximately 35% during our sample period), but probably less than the 63% recidivism rate reported by Kitchener et al. in 1977. With this background, the 52% 25-year recidivism rate implied by the LaGuerre model and the 45 to 49% rate implied by the split lognormal model of this chapter do not seem unreasonable.

Clearly, individuals do differ in their failure rates, and the most failure-prone individuals will tend to fail first. The failure rate in the surviving population will therefore tend to fall over time, as the most failure-prone individuals are successively removed. Models that ignore such heterogeneity should be expected to overpredict long-term recidivism, because they miss the point that only individuals with low failure rates are likely to still be in the surviving population. Split models allow a rather limited type of heterogeneity, in that there are only two types of individuals, and one type has a failure rate of zero. It is possible to consider similar models with two types of individuals, with different failure rates but where neither rate is necessarily zero. Such a model was used by Carr-Hill and Carr-Hill (1972), Harris, Kaylan, and Maltz (1981), and Maltz (1984). Greenberg (1978) suggests that such models be extended to allow for three distinct types of individuals.

An alternative method for recognizing individual differences is to introduce individual characteristics into the model as explanatory variables, so that each individual has a different failure rate. We will consider models that use individual characteristics as explanatory variables in Chapters 6 and 7. However, despite our initial expectations to the contrary, our results in Chapter 7 will show that split models are still useful even when an extensive list of explanatory variables has been used. Of all the models we use in this study, only the split models imply hazard rates that fall fast enough to fit our data well. These results demonstrate the value of combining the two previously existing strands of the criminological literature on survival analysis, as indicated in Chapter 1.

The Split Exponential Model

In this section, we consider the split exponential model. As noted earlier, this model has been considered previously by Maltz and McCleary (1977), and it is featured prominently in Maltz (1984), where it is referred to as "Model M_I." This is the split model in which the distribution of time until recidivism (conditional on ultimate recidivism) is exponential. The likelihood function for this model is given by Equation 5.4 if the density g and the cdf G are replaced by the exponential cdf and density as given by Equations 3.3 and 3.4. The exponential density contains one parameter, θ, so the split exponential distribution contains θ plus the "splitting" parameter δ (the probability of eventual failure).

For 1978, the maximum likelihood estimates of δ and θ are .4088 and .03158; for 1980, they are .4556 and .03248. Thus the model implies an ultimate failure rate of 40–45%, which compares to the failure rate within follow-up of about 35%. The results of previous studies with long follow-ups (cited earlier) suggest that this estimate of the ultimate failure rate is probably too low. Unsurprisingly, the current estimates of the failure rate θ are considerably higher than the estimates reported for the exponential model of Chapter 4. This should be expected because, in the split model, the failure rate is defined only for the subpopulation that will ultimately fail, whereas the model of Chapter 4 has a failure rate that is defined for the entire cohort.

The likelihood values achieved are −3,357.7 for 1978 and −2,974.8 for 1980, as reported in Table 3.2. These values are considerably higher than the likelihood values for the exponential model of Chapter 4 (−3,430.8 and −3,004.5), and are clearly cause to reject the restriction ($\delta = 1$, so that everyone eventually returns to prison) that would convert the split model back into the previous simple model. Indeed, the likelihood values for the split exponential model are higher (for each year) than the likelihood values for the simple Weibull, lognormal, and log-logistic models. However, they are not as large as the likelihood values for the LaGuerre model (−3355.8 and −2973.2). Thus the fit of the split exponential model to the 1978 and 1980 estimation samples is better than the fit of most of the simple models of Chapter 4, but not as good as the fit of the best of those models.[2]

The predicted density from the 1978 split exponential model is displayed in Figure 5.1, and the goodness of fit statistics for 1978 and 1980 are given in Table 3.2. The quality of the predictions is about what one would expect from the comparison of likelihood values in the previous paragraph. The maximum differences between the predicted and the actual cdf are .024 for 1978 and .028 for 1980, and these are in the same ballpark as the values (.020 and .031) for the simple LaGuerre distribution. The overall chi-squared statistics of 115.2 for 1978 and 174.2 for 1980 are also quite similar to the LaGuerre results (118.2 and 172.4, respectively). Thus the split exponential model predicts about as well as the best of the simple models of Chapter 4.

The general pattern of these predictions is also very similar to that of the LaGuerre distribution, as can be seen by comparing Figure 4.2 and 5.1. In terms of density or hazard, there is a clear tendency to overpredict recidivism for the first 2 months or so, followed by some underprediction of recidivism for about the next year. On the other hand, the fit in the tail (past about 15 months) is quite good. In terms of cdf, there is a tendency to underpredict recidivism at first (the first year for 1978 and the first 7

---

[2] This comparison may be a bit misleading, as the best-fitting model of Chapter 4, the LaGuerre model, contains more parameters than the split exponential model.

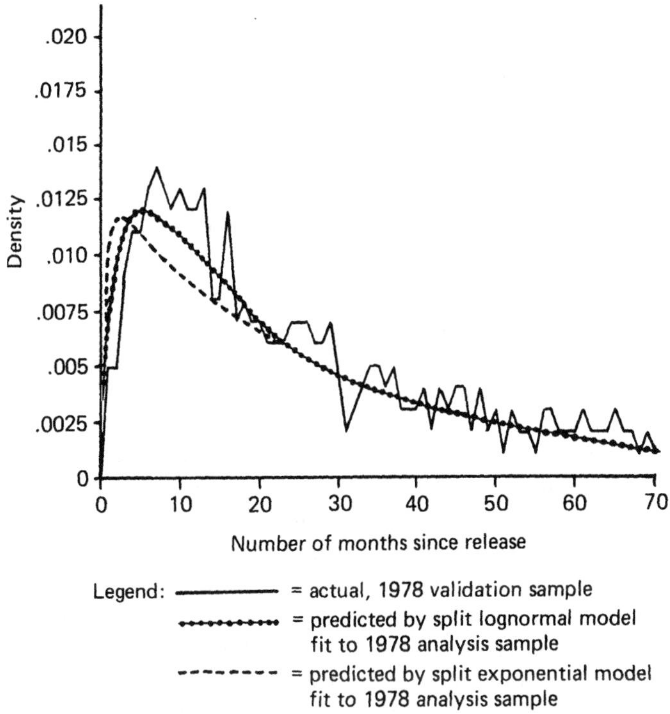

FIGURE 5.1. Predicted versus actual recidivism in the 1978 validation sample: split lognormal and split exponential models.

months for 1980). The remaining predictions are reasonably good for 1978; for 1980, however, there is a noticeable underprediction of recidivism after the first year. Many of the prediction errors (for cdf, density, and hazard) are statistically significantly different from zero, and the rather large overall chi-squared statistics confirm the inadequacy of the model, especially for 1980. Adding the splitting parameter (δ) to our model has clearly helped us to better fit the distribution of the timing of recidivism, but the exponential distribution is still not a good choice.

The Split Lognormal Model

In this section, we consider the split lognormal model. This is the split model in which the distribution of time until recidivism (conditional on eventual recidivism) is lognormal. The likelihood function is again given by Equation 5.4, where the density g and the cdf G are given by Equations 4.1 and 4.2. The parameters to be estimated are the splitting parameter δ and the parameters μ and σ^2 of the lognormal distribution.

The maximum likelihood estimates of δ, μ, and σ^2 are .4477, 3.196, and 1.411 for 1978, and .4929, 3.133, and 1.429 for 1980. The split lognormal model provides the highest values (.45 for 1978 and .49 for 1980) that we will obtain for the splitting parameter (i.e., the ultimate recidivism rate). Given the literature surveyed earlier, these values seem reasonable. Thus it appears that one can expect approximately half of all releasees from North Carolina state prisons to eventually return to them. This is rather depressing but informative. It certainly suggests that any model (including those in the previous chapter) that assumes that all individuals will ultimately fail is far from the mark.

The likelihood values achieved are −3,342.2 for 1978 and −2,955.0 for 1980, as reported in Table 3.2. These likelihood values indicate that the split lognormal distribution fits the 1978 and 1980 estimation samples considerably better than any of the other distributions yet considered.

The results for the split lognormal model's predictions for the 1978 and 1980 validation samples are given in Tables 5.1 and 5.2, and the predicted density for 1978 is displayed as the dotted line in Figure 5.1. These predictions are better than those given by any of the previous parametric models, and they are also better than the nonparametric predictions of Chapter 4. The maximum differences between the predicted and the actual cdf are .005 for 1978 (compared with .020 for the simple LaGuerre model and .012 for the nonparametric model of Chapter 4) and .023 for 1980 (compared with .031 for the simple LaGuerre model and .028 for the nonparametric model of Chapter 4). As can be seen in Table 3.2, these differences are the smallest yet encountered. The overall chi-squared statistics are 50.6 for 1978 and 53.9 for 1980, again the smallest yet encountered. The chi-squared statistics are statistically insignificant at usual confidence levels, indicating that we cannot reject the null hypothesis that the model is correct. The smallest values previously achieved for the chi-squared statistics were for the simple LaGuerre model: 118.2 for 1978 and 172.1 for 1980. Introduction of the splitting parameter has led to a very substantial improvement in the overall fit of our model to our data on the timing of recidivism; it has succeeded in reducing the chi-squared statistics by approximately a factor of three, which is certainly impressive.

Once again, we find that an appropriate parametric model can surpass a nonparametric model markedly in predicting the timing of recidivism. Furthermore, our split models predict markedly better than the corresponding simple models of Chapter 4. It is interesting that our best-fitting model combines the splitting parameter of Anscombe (1961) and Maltz and McCleary (1977) with the lognormal distribution used by Schmidt and Witte (1976, 1978, 1979, 1980, 1984) and Witte and Schmidt (1977). This again illustrates the advantage of combining insights from the different types of work previously done on the timing of recidivism.

Looking at Table 5.1 or Figure 5.1, we can see that the predictions of the split lognormal model for the 1978 data are very satisfactory throughout

TABLE 5.1. Predicted versus actual recidivism rates for 1978 validation sample using split lognormal model fit to 1978 analysis sample.

N	Predicted cdf	cdf	t	Predicted density	Density	t	Predicted hazard	Hazard	t	χ^2	df
0	.000	.000	−.85	.000	.000	−.85	.000	.000	−.85	—	—
1	.004	.005	.85	.004	.005	1.08	.004	.005	1.08	0.7	1
2	.012	.010	−1.29	.008	.005	−2.19	.008	.005	−2.19	5.5	2
3	.023	.019	−1.35	.010	.009	−.59	.011	.010	−.60	5.9	3
4	.035	.031	−1.22	.012	.011	−.20	.012	.012	−.22	5.9	4
5	.047	.042	−1.30	.012	.011	−.47	.013	.012	−.50	6.2	5
6	.059	.055	−1.04	.012	.013	.27	.013	.014	.24	6.2	6
7	.072	.069	−.60	.012	.014	.82	.013	.015	.79	6.8	7
8	.084	.082	−.31	.012	.013	.63	.013	.014	.61	7.2	8
9	.095	.094	−.30	.012	.012	−.02	.013	.013	−.03	7.2	9
10	.107	.107	−.04	.011	.013	.70	.013	.014	.69	7.7	10
11	.118	.119	.15	.011	.012	.59	.012	.013	.59	8.0	11
12	.128	.131	.45	.010	.012	1.02	.012	.014	1.02	9.1	12
13	.138	.144	.86	.010	.013	1.46	.012	.015	1.48	11.3	13
14	.148	.151	.55	.010	.008	−1.04	.011	.009	−1.01	12.3	14
15	.157	.160	.37	.009	.008	−.63	.011	.010	−.61	12.7	15
16	.166	.171	.79	.009	.012	1.71	.010	.014	1.72	15.7	16
17	.174	.178	.59	.008	.007	−.79	.010	.009	−.76	16.2	17
18	.182	.186	.54	.008	.008	−.18	.010	.009	−.15	16.3	18
19	.190	.193	.44	.008	.007	−.38	.009	.009	−.35	16.4	19
20	.198	.200	.35	.007	.007	−.38	.009	.008	−.36	16.5	20
21	.205	.206	.18	.007	.006	−.83	.009	.007	−.82	17.2	21
22	.212	.212	.09	.007	.006	−.43	.009	.008	−.42	17.4	22
23	.218	.218	−.05	.007	.006	−.69	.008	.007	−.69	17.8	23
24	.224	.224	.03	.006	.007	.39	.008	.009	.39	18.0	24
25	.230	.232	.18	.006	.007	.81	.008	.009	.81	18.7	25
26	.236	.239	.35	.006	.007	1.00	.008	.009	1.01	19.7	26
27	.242	.245	.43	.006	.006	.46	.007	.008	.48	19.9	27
28	.247	.251	.49	.005	.006	.39	.007	.008	.41	20.1	28

TABLE 5.1. *Continued*.

N	Predicted cdf	cdf	t	Predicted density	Density	t	Predicted hazard	Hazard	t	χ^2	df
29	.252	.258	.71	.005	.007	1.31	.007	.009	1.34	21.9	29
30	.257	.262	.61	.005	.004	−.57	.007	.006	−.54	22.2	30
31	.262	.264	.29	.005	.002	−2.00	.006	.003	−1.98	26.1	31
32	.266	.267	.04	.005	.003	−1.63	.006	.004	−1.62	28.7	32
33	.271	.271	.02	.004	.004	−.16	.006	.006	−.16	28.7	33
34	.275	.276	.06	.004	.005	.25	.006	.006	.25	28.8	34
35	.279	.280	.11	.004	.005	.39	.006	.006	.39	29.0	35
36	.283	.284	.10	.004	.004	−.05	.005	.005	−.05	29.0	36
37	.287	.288	.19	.004	.005	.65	.005	.006	.66	29.4	37
38	.291	.291	.10	.004	.003	−.70	.005	.004	−.70	29.9	38
39	.294	.295	.06	.004	.003	−.30	.005	.005	−.29	30.0	39
40	.298	.298	−.01	.003	.003	−.50	.005	.004	−.50	30.2	40
41	.301	.301	.02	.003	.004	.23	.005	.005	.23	30.3	41
42	.304	.303	−.13	.003	.002	−1.25	.005	.003	−1.25	31.8	42
43	.307	.307	.00	.003	.004	1.09	.004	.006	1.09	33.0	43
44	.310	.310	−.05	.003	.003	−.43	.004	.004	−.43	33.2	44
45	.313	.314	.03	.003	.004	.66	.004	.005	.66	33.6	45
46	.316	.317	.12	.003	.004	.77	.004	.005	.77	34.2	46
47	.319	.319	.02	.003	.002	−.85	.004	.003	−.84	34.9	47
48	.322	.323	.17	.003	.004	1.33	.004	.006	1.33	36.7	48

49	.324	.325	.13	.003	.002	−.34	.004	.003	−.33	36.8	49
50	.327	.328	.22	.003	.003	.82	.004	.005	.83	37.5	50
51	.329	.329	.04	.002	.001	−1.64	.004	.001	−1.64	40.2	51
52	.331	.332	.07	.002	.003	.27	.004	.004	.27	40.3	52
53	.334	.334	−.01	.002	.002	−.78	.003	.002	−.77	40.9	53
54	.336	.336	−.04	.002	.002	−.33	.003	.003	−.33	41.0	54
55	.338	.337	−.14	.002	.001	−1.03	.003	.002	−1.03	42.0	55
56	.340	.340	.04	.002	.003	.99	.003	.004	.99	43.0	56
57	.342	.342	.02	.002	.003	.68	.003	.004	.68	43.5	57
58	.344	.344	.02	.002	.002	−.05	.003	.003	−.05	43.5	58
59	.346	.346	−.02	.002	.002	−.39	.003	.002	−.39	43.6	59
60	.348	.348	.02	.002	.002	.50	.003	.003	.50	43.9	60
61	.350	.352	.19	.002	.003	1.84	.003	.005	1.84	47.3	61
62	.352	.354	.25	.002	.002	.65	.003	.004	.65	47.7	62
63	.353	.356	.31	.002	.002	.72	.003	.004	.73	48.2	63
64	.355	.358	.34	.002	.002	.35	.003	.003	.36	48.3	64
65	.357	.361	.45	.002	.003	1.30	.003	.004	1.32	50.1	65
66	.358	.363	.52	.002	.002	.93	.002	.004	.94	—	—
67	.360	.365	.53	.002	.002	.08	.002	.003	.10	50.6	66
68	.361	.366	.50	.002	.001	−.32	.002	.002	−.31	—	—
69	.363	.367	.52	.001	.002	.20	.002	.003	.21	50.6	67
70	.364	.369	.50	.001	.001	.22	.002	.002	−.21	—	—

TABLE 5.2. Predicted versus actual recidivism rates for 1980 validation sample using split lognormal model fit to 1980 analysis sample.

N	Predicted cdf	cdf	t	Predicted density	Density	t	Predicted hazard	Hazard	t	χ^2	df
0	.000	.001	3.77	.000	.001	3.77	.000	.001	3.77	—	—
1	.006	.005	−.80	.005	.003	−1.79	.005	.003	−1.78	0.6	1
2	.016	.014	−.81	.010	.010	−.41	.010	.010	−.42	0.8	2
3	.029	.030	.47	.013	.016	1.59	.013	.016	1.58	3.3	3
4	.043	.046	1.16	.014	.016	1.33	.015	.017	1.34	5.1	4
5	.057	.064	1.88	.015	.018	1.68	.015	.019	1.71	8.0	5
6	.072	.079	1.88	.015	.015	.40	.015	.016	.46	8.2	6
7	.086	.094	1.74	.014	.014	.03	.015	.016	.09	8.2	7
8	.100	.111	2.39	.014	.017	1.95	.015	.019	2.02	12.3	8
9	.114	.126	2.60	.013	.015	.94	.015	.017	1.04	13.4	9
10	127	.141	2.96	.013	.015	1.40	.015	.018	1.52	15.7	10
11	.139	.157	3.40	.012	.015	1.75	.014	.018	1.90	19.3	11
12	.151	.171	3.76	.012	.014	1.56	.014	.017	1.73	22.3	12
13	.162	.183	3.66	.011	.011	.05	.013	.014	.22	22.3	13
14	.173	.194	3.63	.011	.011	.23	.013	.014	.40	22.5	14
15	.183	.205	3.74	.010	.011	.71	.012	.014	.89	23.3	15
16	.193	.214	3.54	.010	.009	−.51	.012	.011	−.34	23.4	16
17	.202	.224	3.54	.009	.010	.26	.012	.012	.43	23.6	17
18	.211	.234	3.61	.009	.010	.56	.011	.013	.74	24.1	18
19	.220	.240	3.20	.009	.006	−1.62	.011	.008	−1.47	26.3	19
20	.228	.249	3.33	.008	.009	.82	.010	.012	.99	27.3	20
21	.236	.257	3.34	.008	.008	.24	.010	.011	.40	27.4	21

22	.243	.262	2.84	.007	.004	−2.33	.010	.006	−2.20	32.3	22
23	.250	.269	2.78	.007	.007	−.14	.009	.009	−.01	32.3	23
24	.257	.274	2.53	.007	.005	−1.20	.009	.007	−1.08	33.5	24
25	.264	.282	2.64	.007	.007	.71	.009	.010	.84	34.2	25
26	.270	.287	2.55	.006	.006	−.40	.009	.008	−.28	34.2	26
27	.276	.294	2.60	.006	.007	.40	.008	.009	.52	34.5	27
28	.282	.298	2.35	.006	.004	−1.39	.008	.006	−1.29	36.2	28
29	.288	.303	2.20	.006	.005	−.81	.008	.007	−.71	36.7	29
30	.293	.307	1.99	.005	.004	−1.26	.008	.006	−1.17	38.0	30
31	.298	.311	1.87	.005	.004	−.67	.007	.006	−.58	38.4	31
32	.303	.318	2.12	.005	.007	1.68	.007	.010	1.78	41.6	32
33	.308	.322	2.03	.005	.004	−.55	.007	.006	−.46	41.8	33
34	.312	.327	2.10	.005	.005	.51	.007	.008	.61	42.1	34
35	.317	.334	2.38	.004	.007	2.07	.006	.010	2.19	46.9	35
36	.321	.338	2.40	.004	.004	.16	.006	.007	.27	47.0	36
37	.325	.340	2.14	.004	.002	−1.83	.006	.004	−1.75	50.1	37
38	.329	.344	2.03	.004	.003	−.74	.006	.005	−.65	50.5	38
39	.333	.348	2.05	.004	.004	.14	.006	.006	.23	50.5	39
40	.337	.351	2.01	.004	.003	−.22	.006	.005	−.14	50.5	40
41	.340	.354	1.96	.004	.003	−.34	.005	.005	−.26	50.6	41
42	.344	.357	1.84	.003	.003	−1.00	.005	.004	−.92	51.5	42
43	.347	.360	1.85	.003	.003	.17	.005	.005	.25	51.5	43
44	.350	.362	1.69	.003	.002	−1.31	.005	.003	−1.25	53.1	44
45	.353	.365	1.58	.003	.002	−.94	.005	.004	.88	53.9	45
46	.356	.368	1.55	.003	.003	−.28	.005	.004	−.21	53.9	46

the whole range of the distribution, and this is true whether we consider predictions of the cdf, density, or hazard. The prediction errors are almost all insignificantly different from zero (at usual confidence levels), and the only noticeable pattern is a slight tendency to overpredict recidivism for the first 6 months or so (especially the predictions of the cdf) and to underpredict recidivism for a few months thereafter. Simply put, the model seems to fit the data adequately.

On the other hand, looking at Table 5.2, we see that the model's predictions for the 1980 data are somewhat less satisfactory. In terms of cdf, the model underpredicts recidivism for virtually all lengths of time after release. In terms of density or hazard, the model underpredicts recidivism for the first 18 or 20 months and overpredicts very slightly thereafter. These predictive errors follow (to a lesser extent) the same general pattern as was found in the 1980 nonparametric predictions. Apparently, the errors simply reflect the fact that the recidivism rate is higher in the 1980 validation sample than in the 1980 estimation sample. Given that fact, there is obviously some limit as to how well any model fit to the 1980 estimation sample can be expected to predict for the 1980 validation sample.

Overall, the performance of the split lognormal model is quite encouraging. Its predictions are better than the nonparametric predictions, showing the potential advantage of using a parametric model. It performs better than any of the simple models of the previous chapter, and indeed (as can be seen in Table 3.2) it performs better than any of the other split models of this chapter. Further, as we will show in Chapter 7, this model predicts as well as our best model that includes explanatory variables. This is somewhat surprising, because it indicates that those seeking to predict only for *random samples of releasees* might just as well use the split lognormal model of this section as the more sophisticated models of Chapter 7.

The Split Log-Logistic Model

The split log-logistic model is the split model in which the distribution of time until recidivism (conditional on eventual recidivism) is log-logistic. The likelihood function is of the form of Equation 5.4, with the log-logistic density g and cdf G given by Equations 4.3 and 4.4. The parameters to be estimated are the splitting parameter δ and the parameters α and k of the log-logistic distribution.

The maximum likelihood estimates of δ, α, and k are .4318, .04342, and 1.523 for 1978, and .4654, .04793, and 1.501 for 1980. The estimates for the splitting parameter (δ) and for k are quite interesting. Note that the values for the splitting parameter are lower than the values for the split lognormal model of the previous section. Indeed, they seem a bit too low to be reasonable, given what we know about the ultimate rate of return to prison for releasees. The values of k achieved for the split log-logistic model are far higher than the values achieved for the simple log-logistic model of Chapter 4. Recall from Chapter 4 that the hazard rate is monotonic if $k < 1$ and has a single maximum if $k > 1$. As our data have a single maximum, we would expect to obtain values of k greater than one. We did not obtain such values in Chapter 4; however, we do obtain them here. This fact again provides evidence of the usefulness of the splitting parameter for models of the timing of recidivism.

The likelihood values achieved are −3,340.6 for 1978 and −2,958.8 for 1980, as reported in Table 3.2. These are rather similar to the corresponding values for the split lognormal model (−3,342.2 and −2,955.0 respectively). The split log-logistic model fits the 1978 estimation sample slightly better than the split lognormal model does, but it fits the 1980 estimation sample slightly worse.

The predictions of the split log-logistic model for the 1978 and 1980 validation samples are fairly good, but not quite as good as the corresponding predictions for the split lognormal model. As can be seen in Table 3.2, the maximum differences between the predicted and the actual cdf are .011 for 1978 and .024 for 1980, which are larger than the corresponding values (.005 and .023) for the split lognormal model. Similarly, the overall chi-squared statistics are 61.0 for 1978 and 76.4 for 1980. These are slightly larger than the corresponding split lognormal values (50.6 and 53.9, respectively).

The predictions of the split log-logistic model for the 1978 validation sample are quite good, with very few statistically significant prediction errors. However, the split log-logistic model fits slightly less well than the split lognormal for months three through twelve (where it tends to underpredict recidivism) and in the tail of the distribution (where it again tends to underpredict recidivism). The model's predictions for the 1980 validation sample are less satisfactory than those for 1978, as expected. The pattern of the prediction errors is rather similar to that of the prediction errors for the split lognormal model, as described in the last section, but the fit is worse, especially for the first year or so after release.

The performance of the split log-logistic model is thus reasonably satisfactory. However, the split lognormal model is slightly superior.

The Split Weibull Model

The split Weibull model is the split model in which the distribution of time until recidivism (conditional on eventual recidivism) is Weibull. The likelihood function is again given by Equation 5.4 but with the density g and cdf G given by Equations 4.6 and 4.7. The parameters to be estimated are the splitting parameter δ and the parameters θ and k of the Weibull distribution.

The maximum likelihood estimates of δ, θ, and k are .3840, .03537, and 1.238 for 1978, and .3997, .04135, and 1.267 for 1980. The estimated values of the ultimate recidivism rate (δ) seem unreasonably low. Also note that the estimate of k exceeds one for both years and indicates an *increasing* hazard rate for the population of ultimate failures (see the section The Weibull Model, Chapter 4.) This is apparently necessary to improve the fit of the distribution to the very early part of our data, where the hazard rate does indeed increase. The "split" nature of the model implies that the hazard rate for the entire population will ultimately decrease, so as to match the decrease in the hazard rate in the rest of our data (past the first few months). However, this decrease in the predicted hazard rate comes too late for the model to fit adequately.

The likelihood values achieved are −3,346.2 for 1978 and −2,964.1 for 1980, as reported in Table 3.2. As might be expected, these are lower than for the split lognormal or split log-logistic models, indicating a poorer fit of the model to the estimation samples. Similarly, the predictions of the model for the 1978 and 1980 validation samples are also not as good as those given by the split lognormal and split log-logistic models. The maximum differences between the predicted and actual cdf's are .017 for 1978 and .032 for 1980, while the overall chi-squared statistics are 95.9 and 118.5, as can be seen in Table 3.2. The chi-squared statistics are approximately double the values achieved by the split lognormal model. For both years, the model overpredicts recidivism for the period immediately after release, underpredicts recidivism for the next year or so, and then fits reasonably well in the tail.

Overall, the split Weibull model is more adequate than any of our simple models of Chapter 4 and is also better than the split exponential model (or the split LaGuerre model, to be considered in the next section). However, it is not as adequate as the split lognormal and split log-logistic models.

The Split LaGuerre Model

The split LaGuerre model is the split model in which the distribution of time until recidivism (conditional on eventual recidivism) is LaGuerre. The LaGuerre model was the best of our simple models of Chapter 4, but the split LaGuerre model does not compare as favorably with the other split models of this chapter.

The likelihood function is again given by Equation 5.4, where the density g and cdf G are given by Equations 4.9 and 4.10. The parameters to be estimated are the splitting parameter δ and the parameters α, δ_1, and δ_2 for the LaGuerre distribution. The maximum likelihood estimates of δ, α, δ_1, and δ_2 are .3825, .06698, 2.8661, and .007049 for 1978, and .3953, .08232, 3.974, and .008303 for 1980. Note that the values for the splitting parameters imply an ultimate rate of recidivism that is unreasonably low.

The likelihood values achieved are −3,349.1 for 1978 and −2,967.6 for 1980, as can be seen in Table 3.2. These are larger (indicating a better fit) than for any of our simple models but smaller than for any of our other split models except the split exponential. More or less the same story is told by the model's predictions for the 1978 and 1980 validation samples. The maximum differences between the predicted and actual cdf's are .021 for 1978 and .034 for 1980, while the overall chi-squared statistics are 113.8 and 133.0 as reported in Table 3.2. These values are larger (indicating less satisfactory predictions) than for any of the other split models except the split exponential. This model gives us the familiar pattern of overprediction of recidivism for the first few months after release, followed by a period of underprediction of recidivism. Compared to our more successful models, however, the magnitude of the prediction errors is larger for the split LaGuerre model, and the period of underprediction is longer. The conclusion is simple. Introduction of the splitting parameter allows alternative parametric models to outperform the LaGuerre. This was not the case for the simple models, with no splitting parameter, of Chapter 4.

Conclusions

In this chapter, we have considered split population models of the type introduced by Maltz and McCleary (1977). These models contain a parameter (the so-called "splitting parameter") that represents the probability that an individual would ultimately return to prison. The value of this probability may be of interest to criminal justice researchers and practitioners. For criminal justice researchers, it provides an estimate of the proportion of releasees who "drop out" of crime, a central feature of career criminal research, where it is called the "termination rate." For practitioners, it may provide useful information for projecting future prison populations or for assessing the likely incapacitative effect of incarceration or the effectiveness of alternative correctional treatments (e.g., management styles, security levels, programming).

Our use of split population models was quite successful in terms of providing a good fit to our estimation samples and good predictions for our validation samples. Compared with the simple models of Chapter 4, the split models of this chapter fit the estimation samples better, and they resulted in better predictions for the validation samples. Indeed, the *worst* of our split models (the split exponential) was about as good as the *best* of the simple models (the LaGuerre).

This is especially striking since the split exponential model actually contains fewer parameters than the LaGuerre model, and our best split models contain the same number of parameters as the LaGuerre model. In any statistical model, there is the potential to improve the fit by adding another parameter. Apparently, the "splitting parameter" is a good canadidate for early inclusion. This is certainly true in our data, and it is likely to be so in other data sets in which the hazard rate falls sharply with time since release. Split models will generally imply rapidly falling hazard rates, because they imply that the surviving population is increasingly made up of individuals with zero failure rates. Thus split models will tend to provide a good fit to data sets with this same characteristic.

Our best model so far is the split lognormal model. Its predictions for the 1978 validation sample are very satisfactory. Its predictions for the 1980 validation sample are less so, but they are probably as good as can be expected, given the difference in recidivism rates between the 1980 estimation and validation samples.

In the next two chapters, we will consider models that use individual characteristics as explanatory variables. These models introduce heterogeneity of individuals in a different way than split models do, but they share the important feature of implying a rapidly decreasing hazard rate (after a short initial period of increase). We will find many individual characteristics that are significantly related to recidivism, but we will not find a model that provides better predictions for our validation samples than the split lognormal model of this chapter. Rather, the potential usefulness of models with explanatory variables lies in their ability to make predictions for nonrandomly chosen subpopulations and for individuals.

6
The Proportional Hazards Model

Introduction

In this chapter and Chapter 7, we will consider models of the length of time until recidivism that contain individual characteristics as explanatory variables. The models of Chapter 7 will be parametric models in the sense that they will assume a particular distribution for the survival times; for example, we will estimate a model based on the exponential distribution, in which the mean of the distribution depends on individual characteristics. In this chapter, on the other hand, we will consider the proportional hazards model of Cox (1972). This model allows one to estimate the effects of individual characteristics on survival times without having to assume a particular form for the distribution function (or the density or hazard). Instead, the distribution of the survival times is estimated in a nonparametric way. This model has been used a good deal recently in the study of recidivism. For example, see Barton and Turnbull (1981), Rhodes and Matsuba (1985), Sherman and Berk (1984), and Witte et al. (1982).

Our main interest in the proportional hazards analysis is to determine which individual characteristics have significant effects on length of time until recidivism, without making a specific distributional assumption. This is of interest in its own right, and it will also be useful in deciding which individual characteristics are worth entering into our parametric models of Chapter 7. The "goodness of fit" of the nonparametric proportional hazards model will also provide a benchmark for judging the parametric models of Chapter 7.

The Model and Its Estimation

For an individual with a (row) vector **X** of demographic (or other) characteristics, the proportional hazards model assumes a hazard rate of the form:

$$h(t|\mathbf{X}) = h_0(t)e^{\mathbf{X}\beta}, \tag{6.1}$$

where $h_0(t)$ is a completely unspecified "baseline" hazard function. Thus the model assumes that the hazard functions of any two individuals differ only by a factor of proportionality, but it puts no further restrictions on these hazard functions.

The vector $\boldsymbol{\beta}$ shows the direction of effect of the various elements of $\mathbf{X}$ (the various individual characteristics) on the hazard rate. For example, a positive element of $\boldsymbol{\beta}$ indicates that an increase in the corresponding variable in $\mathbf{X}$ will increase the hazard rate and thus will (on average) reduce the length of time until recidivism. As indicated earlier, the point of the model is to estimate $\boldsymbol{\beta}$ without making any assumptions (beyond the proportionality assumption) about the form of the hazard function.

We will estimate $\boldsymbol{\beta}$ by maximizing the *partial likelihood function* proposed by Cox (1975). To define the partial likelihood, suppose that the sample consists of N individuals and that n of these individuals fail (return to prison) before the end of the follow-up period. Index these failures by $i = 1, 2, \ldots, n$; the nonfailures are therefore indexed by $i = n + 1, \ldots, N$. Suppose that individual i fails at time t_i. For any time t, define $R(t)$ as the set of all $i = 1, \ldots, N$ such that individual i was still at risk (had not yet failed) just prior to time t. In particular, for any observed failure time t_i, $R(t_i)$ includes recidivists whose failure times are at least of length t_i, as well as those nonrecidivists whose follow-up times are at least of length t_i.

For any observed failure time t_i, the probability that it is individual i who should fail (given that exactly one individual from the set $R(t_i)$ fails at that time) is given by:

$$h(t_i|\mathbf{X}_i) / \sum_{j \in R(t_i)} h(t_i|\mathbf{X}_j) = e^{\mathbf{X}_i\boldsymbol{\beta}} / \sum_{j \in R(t_i)} e^{\mathbf{X}_j\boldsymbol{\beta}}. \tag{6.2}$$

The partial likelihood function is then formed by multiplying Equation 6.2 over all n failure times:

$$L = \prod_{i=1}^{n} \{e^{\mathbf{X}_i\boldsymbol{\beta}} / \sum_{j \in R(t_i)} e^{\mathbf{X}_j\boldsymbol{\beta}}\}. \tag{6.3}$$

A problem that often arises in practice, and that does arise in our data, is that there may be "ties," in the sense that more than one individual may have the same reported failure time. For example, in the 1978 estimation sample, 24 individuals have TIME = 15 months, and it is obvious that such ties arise because we have rounded the time until recidivism to the nearest month. This is a problem because the partial likelihood of Equation 6.3 was derived under the assumption that only one individual failed at any point in time. The correct partial likelihood in the presence of ties is very complicated; for example, see Kalbfleisch and Prentice (1980, equation 4.7, p. 74). We adopt the approximation suggested by Peto (1972), which was reported also by Kalbfleisch and Prentice (1980, Equation 4.8, p. 74) and which amounts to simply using Equation 6.3 despite the occurrence of ties.[1] This approximation is thought to be satisfactory if the proportion of the failures that occur at any point in time is small, and this is true in our case.

Results of Estimation

The results of our estimation of the proportional hazards model are given in Table 6.1 for the 1978 analysis sample and in Table 6.2 for the 1980 analysis sample. We began with an original specification which included the 15 explanatory variables defined in Chapter 2: TSERVD, AGE, PRIORS, RULE, SCHOOL, WHITE, MALE, ALCHY, JUNKY, MARRIED, SUPER, WORKREL, FELON, PERSON, and PROPTY. (In order to make the sizes of the coefficients more nearly equal, however, some of these variables were rescaled; for example, AGE/1,000 measures age in thousands of months, rather than in single months. This is purely a matter of convenience and has no substantive implications whatsoever.)

As pointed out by Farrington and Tarling (1985), the ideal way of selecting explanatory variables would be on the basis of a fully developed theory. As economists, we are certainly sympathetic to this position. However, as numerous researchers have pointed out, the current state of criminological theory is not strong.[2] Furthermore, our choice of explanatory variables was constrained by the data we had available. Our data contain considerable information on the demographic characteristics of the individuals and on the individuals' prior criminal records. However, our data do not contain information on environmental factors (such as economic conditions, policies of the criminal justice system, or opportunities to commit crimes) that might affect the criminal decision. We searched previous empirical work to identify important factors affecting criminality, and the explanatory variables that we used are seen as important in the literature. We fail to include a number of factors that were found to be important in previous research because they are not available in our data. For example, our data do not include information on childhood experiences,[3]

[1] Note that Barton and Turnbull (1981) have discussed and used a similar approximation.

[2] For example, see Martin, Sechrest, and Redner (1981) or Wilson and Herrnstein (1985). Two interesting trends are appearing in the development of criminological theory. The first is well represented by the work of Wilson and Herrnstein who develop an eclectic model that draws on the insights of numerous theories and the findings of inductive studies. The second trend can be found in the work of Tauchen, Tauchen, and Witte (1986) and Flinn (1986). These authors seek to develop formal stochastic, dynamic models of criminal behavior.

[3] See Blumstein et al. (1986, vol. 1, chap. 2) or Wilson and Herrnstein (1985, chap. 8).

TABLE 6.1. Proportional hazards model, 1978 analysis sample.

Variable	Final specification		Original specification	
	Coefficient	t ratio	Coefficient	t ratio
TSERVD/100	1.37120	8.15	1.1620000	5.92
AGE/1,000	−3.49690	−7.09	−3.3445000	−6.43
PRIORS/10	.89883	6.75	.8360200	6.09
WHITE	−.44041	−5.07	−.4447500	−5.07
FELON	−.57342	−4.10	−.5786600	−3.54
ALCHY	.41250	3.98	.4285000	4.11
JUNKY	.31512	3.28	.2820400	2.91
PROPTY	.40483	3.02	.3901200	2.47
MALE	.70252	2.92	.6756900	2.78
RULE/100			3.0861000	1.83
MARRIED			−.1529000	−1.42
SCHOOL/10			−.2508200	−1.29
WORKREL			.0860480	.96
PERSON			.0755440	.31
SUPER			−.0087688	−.09
ln L	−3,970.7		3,967.0	

TABLE 6.2. Proportional hazards model, 1980 analysis sample.

Variable	Final specification		Original specification	
	Coefficient	t ratio	Coefficient	t ratio
PRIORS/10	.98466	8.95	.95161	8.44
TSERVD/100	1.13140	−7.47	1.05300	−5.97
AGE/1,000	−3.87610	−6.54	−3.95250	−6.46
ALCHY	.36354	3.80	.35561	3.68
PROPTY	.32162	3.53	.35834	3.31
MARRIED	−.39381	−3.17	−.40394	−3.21
WHITE	−.23783	−2.68	−.25432	−2.82
JUNKY	.23895	2.37	.24305	2.38
MALE	.56221	2.20	.52635	2.05
SCHOOL/10			−.38496	−1.78
WORKREL			.13737	1.45
RULE/100			1.90240	1.43
FELON			−.13378	−1.30
SUPER			.10588	.95
PERSON			−.11739	−.69
ln L	−3,634.1		−3,629.4	

age of initiation of criminal activity,[4] or whether the individual lived in a rural or urban area.[5] However, our specification does include measures of most major factors believed to affect recidivism.

[4] See Blumstein et al. (1986, vol. 1, chap. 3) or Wilson and Herrnstein (1985, chap. 5).

[5] See Wilson and Herrnstein (1985, chap. 11).

The results for this specification are given in Tables 6.1 and 6.2, under the heading Original Specification. We give the coefficients (the elements of β, in the notation of the last section) for each variable, as well as the asymptotic "t ratio" for each coefficient. These t ratios are asymptotically distributed as standard normal, under the null hypothesis that the corresponding coefficient equals zero.

For each year, nine of the variables have coefficients that are significantly different from zero at the 5% level (as indicated by t ratios in excess of 1.96 in absolute value), and six do not. For each year, we reached a final specification by dropping the six variables whose coefficients were insignificantly different from zero in the original specification.[6] The results for this specification are also given in Tables 6.1 and 6.2, under the heading Final Specification.

The results for 1978 (Table 6.1) and for 1980 (Table 6.2) are remarkably similar. Five of the six variables that had statistically insignificant coefficients were the same in both years: RULE, SCHOOL, WORKREL, PERSON, and SUPER. (The coefficient of FELON was significant in 1978 but insignificant in 1980, whereas the coefficient of MARRIED was significant in 1980 but insignificant in 1978.) All coefficients that are significant in either year are of the same sign for both years. Most coefficients are of about the same magnitude for both years. The three variables that are the most significant (as measured by their t ratios) are the same for both years: TSERVD, AGE, and PRIORS. These results are also broadly consistent with the findings of previous studies.[7]

Our results indicate that the type of individual most likely to return to prison (and most likely to have a *small* value of time until recidivism) is a young, black male with a large number of previous incarcerations, who is a drug addict and/or alcoholic, and whose previous incarceration was lengthy and for a crime against property. On the other hand, our results indicate that an individual's likelihood of recidivism is not significantly affected by the following factors: the extent of formal education, the number of prison rule violations, participation in the North Carolina prisoner work release

---

[6] We also performed a likelihood ratio test of the joint significance of these variables. The test statistic is twice the difference of the log-likelihood values, with the variables first included and then dropped. This test statistic equals 7.4 for 1978 and 9.4 for 1980, and in both cases is insignificant at the 5% level. (The appropriate asymptotic distribution under the null hypothesis that all six coefficients equal zero is chi-squared, with six degrees of freedom.) It is important to test the joint significance of the variables before dropping them. This ensures that their individual insignificance is not just the result of multicollinearity.

[7] For previous work on recidivism in North Carolina, see Service (1972), Schmidt and Witte (1976, 1978, 1979, 1980, 1984), and Witte and Schmidt (1977). For more general surveys, see Monahan (1981), Wilson and Herrnstein (1985), Farrington and Tarling (1985), and Blumstein et al. (1986).

program, release from the previous incarceration under supervision, and whether or not the previous incarceration was for a crime against a person.

These findings, with the possible exception of the findings on race, are consistent with the conclusions of one of the two most comprehensive surveys available (Wilson & Herrnstein, 1985), with some of the conclusions of the second such survey (Blumstein et al., 1986) and our own previous work (Schmidt & Witte, 1984). Wilson and Herrnstein (1985) conclude that crime is a young man's game, and this is certainly consistent with our findings. In another comprehensive survey, Wish and Johnson (1986, p.53) conclude that "as levels of illicit drug use increase so does criminal activity." Collins (1986) reaches a similar conclusion regarding alcohol use and criminality.[8] The National Academy of Sciences' Panel on Research on Criminal Careers concludes that "high rates of criminal activity in the past are a good indication of continued future offending at high frequencies" (Blumstein et al., 1986, vol. 1, p. 75). This is certainly consistent with our findings regarding previous criminal record.

Our findings regarding the relationship between race and recidivism are more controversial. Indeed, in our own previous work using data on 1969 and 1971 releasees, we found *whites* more likely to be rearrested (Schmidt & Witte, 1984), which is the opposite of our current finding. After a careful survey of a broad range of literature on the relationship between race and crime, Wilson and Herrnstein (1985, p. 461) conclude, "Even allowing for the existence of discriminatiion in the criminal justice system, the higher rates of crimes among black Americans cannot be denied." Wilson and Herrnstein suggest various possible explanations for the difference in crime rates between whites and blacks (constitutional factors, economic deprivation, a "culture of poverty," and a "subculture of violence"), but they conclude that the existing empirical evidence does not allow one to identify the source of the black/white differential in crime rates. The recent report of the Panel on Research on Criminal Careers reaches a somewhat different conclusion. The panel concludes that sex, age, and race affect the probability of participation in crime but not the frequency with which offenses occur (Blumstein et al., 1976, p. 76). At this point, we are not able to resolve this controversy because the proportional hazards model does not allow us to distinguish the effects of explanatory variables on the participation decision from their effects on frequency of offending. However, some of the models we consider in Chapter 7 do allow us to make this distinction, and we will return to this issue when these models are discussed.

---

[8] It should be noted that there is some controversy regarding the direction of causation between drug or alcohol use and crime. See Blumstein et al. (1986, vol. 1).

Predictions From the Proportional Hazards Model

We now use the proportional hazards model, estimated using the 1978 and 1980 estimation samples, to predict the recidivism rates in the corresponding validation samples. This requires, first of all, that we estimate the baseline hazard function $h_0(t)$, as in the section The Model and Its Estimation. Once we have estimated the baseline hazard, we can construct the hazard function of each individual in the sample according to Equation 6.1; for individual i, simply use the appropriate vector $\mathbf{X}_i$ of characteristics. Given the hazard function for each individual, we can then construct the density and cumulative distribution function, and the model's predictions follow as in the section Predictions Using Survival Time Models (Chapter 3).

To estimate the baseline hazard function, it is necessary to recognize that the apparently discrete nature of our dependent variable (TIME) is due to rounding the length of time until return to prison to the nearest month. The discrete model that arises from grouping (rounding) of time in the continuous-time model is discussed by Kalbfleisch and Prentice (1980, section 4.6). The appropriate likelihood function is also given (Kalbfleisch & Prentice, 1980, equation 4.32, p. 99). This likelihood function depends on $\boldsymbol{\beta}$ and the parameters of the baseline hazard; the number of parameters in the baseline hazard function is the number of possible values that the failure time may take (in our data, 82 for 1978 and 58 for 1980). We can simplify matters considerably by estimating $\boldsymbol{\beta}$ from the continuous-time model, as discussed earlier in this chapter, and using the likelihood of the discrete model to estimate only the parameters of the baseline hazard function. In this case, each of the parameters of the baseline hazard function can be estimated (*separately*) by solving a single nonlinear equation (Kalbfleisch & Prentice, 1980, equation 4.33, p. 99). This is time-consuming, because of the large number of such parameters, but computationally feasible.

The baseline hazard corresponds to the hazard when $\mathbf{X} = 0$, which is an uninteresting (indeed impossible) set of individual characteristics. However, we generated predictions of recidivism by multiplying the baseline hazard by the sample mean values of $e^{\mathbf{X}\boldsymbol{\beta}}$ (which are .877 for 1978 and .901 for 1980). The resulting hazard should correspond at least roughly to the "mean" hazard in the sample. The predictions implied by this "mean" hazard rate are very similar to the nonparametric predictions of Chapter 4. This similarity is certainly not surprising, given the nonparametric nature of the estimation of the distribution of failure times in the proportional hazards model.

A more satisfactory method of prediction, however, is to use the appropriate (individual-specific) hazard function for each individual and to aggregate the individual predictions as indicated in Chapter 3. The results are still very similar to the nonparametric results of Chapter 4, as can be seen from the goodness of fit statistics given in Table 3.2. For example, the maximum differences between the predicted and the actual cdf are .012 for 1978 and .034 for 1980, compared to .012 and .028 for the nonparametric predictions of Chapter 4. The overall chi-squared statistics are 127.1 for 1978 and 232.4 for 1980, and these again are rather similar to the values of Chapter 4 (130.3 and 222.2).

The use of individual characteristics as explanatory variables, therefore, does not improve the quality of our nonparametric predictions, at least not when we are making predictions for a random sample of releasees and are using a model estimated on data from a random sample of releasees. However, as we will see in Chapter 8, models (like the proportional hazards model) that include explanatory variables certainly allow one to make improved predictions for samples of releasees whose characteristics differ from those of the estimation sample. For example, we will see that virtually all of the difference between the 1978 and 1980 recidivism rates is explainable by differences in the (observable) characteristics of the release cohorts. Such a conclusion is obviously not possible without considering models that have explanatory variables.

Conclusions

We have estimated the proportional hazards model using data from the 1978 and 1980 estimation samples. The results, which are quite similar for both years, indicate that the type of individual most likely to return to prison is a young, black male who is a drug addict and/or alcoholic, who has a large number of previous incarcerations, and whose previous incarceration was lengthy and for a crime against property.

We will obtain very similar results using parametric models (exponential and lognormal) in the next chapter. The advantages of the proportional hazards model are that it is easier to estimate than the parametric models, it rests on weaker assumptions, and suitable software can be found in such readily available statistical packages as SAS and BMDP. These advantages make the proportional hazards model a reasonable starting point before going on to more complicated models.

In terms of predicting recidivism, the proportional hazards model suffers from the same defect as the nonparametric "model" of Chapter 4. There is too much month to month variability in the predicted failure rate. A parametric model will "smooth" these predictions, and (just as in Chapter 5) an adequate parametric model can be expected to predict better than any nonparametric model.

7
Parametric Models With Explanatory Variables

Introduction

In this chapter, we consider parametric statistical models that contain individual characteristics as explanatory variables. The explanatory variables that we use are the same as those used for estimating the proportional hazards model in the last chapter. Our estimates of the effects of these explanatory variables on time until recidivism turn out to be very similar to the estimates from the proportional hazards model. However, the parametric models of this chapter impose much more structure on the form of the distribution of time until recidivism than the proportional hazards model did. Accordingly, they lead to rather different predictions of recidivism than those of the proportional hazards model.

We consider models based on the exponential, lognormal, and LaGuerre distributions. We allow these to be split models (in the sense of Chapter 5), and we allow the explanatory variables to affect both the probability of eventual recidivism and the distribution of time until recidivism for those who will eventually return to prison. Although models of this type have not been used previously in survival analyses (as far as we are aware), they are a natural extension of existing models. In particular, they can be viewed as a combination of the two types of models previously used in survival analyses in criminal justice. Following the work of Maltz (1984) and his colleagues, these models do not assume that everyone will eventually fail (i.e., they incorporate a splitting parameter to represent the probability of eventual failure). Following our own earlier work, these models allow explanatory variables to affect the timing of recidivism. However, the innovative aspect of these models is that they also allow explanatory variables to affect the splitting parameter.

The results we obtain using these models are not terribly strong; we have trouble distinguishing the effects of explanatory variables on the probability of eventual recidivism from their effects on the timing of recidivism. What is interesting is that it turns out to be easier to find significant determinants of the probability of eventual recidivism than to find determinants of the timing of recidivism.

Our results may be interpreted in terms of the career criminal paradigm. As noted earlier, the termination rate is simply one minus our probability of eventual recidivism. The frequency of offending is directly related to the timing of offenses, which we model directly for those who do not terminate their careers after release from prison. Previous work on termination (see Blumstein et al., 1986, chap. 3) has suggested that a number of personal characteristics are associated with termination. However, this work has not explicitly allowed for the censoring of information on offending, which casts some doubt on the validity of the results. We explicitly account for the censoring in our data and, further, simultaneously model both the probability of continuing in crime and the timing of new offenses for those who persist in crime. Like the existing literature, we are far more successful in finding correlates of persistence than we are in finding correlates for the frequency of offending.

Future studies of recidivism that rely on data with a larger set of explanatory variables may be more successful than our study was in distinguishing the factors related to the probability of recidivism from the factors related to its timing. As noted by Blumstein et al. (1986), an ability to make such distinctions could be very important both for our understanding of criminality and for criminal justice policy. For example, identifying a set of factors associated with termination could help the criminal justice system to better use both its rehabilitative resources and its prison space. Identifying a set of factors related to timing could help us better understand the "career criminal."

However, the methodology we develop has potentially broader use. It may be used not only to study the termination probability and frequency of offending for offenders, but also with data bases for general population groups to study simultaneously the factors affecting the probability of ever participating in criminal activity and the timing of offenses for those who do participate. The recent report of the Panel on Research on Criminal Careers (Blumstein et al., 1986) suggests that the probability of offending and the timing of offenses for those who do offend are determined by quite different factors. Our methodology would provide a very useful test of this contention.

There are a number of existing data bases that might be used to test the Panel's hypothesis using our methodology.[1] Further, there have recently been a number of proposals for collecting new, large longitudinal data bases that would contain information on criminal activity as well as a large range of potential explanatory variables. For example, see Blumstein et al. (1986) or Farrington et al. (1986). Indeed the Office of Juvenile

[1] See Farrington (1979), Blumstein et al. (1986, vol. 1), or Farrington et al. (1986) for a survey and description of available data sets. Perhaps the most famous and widely-used of these data sets are the two Philadelphia cohorts studied by Wolfgang and his colleagues (e.g., Tracy, Wolfgang, & Figlio, 1985).

Justice and Delinquency Prevention has recently funded preliminary work on some new longitudinal data bases. Such data sets with extensive information on each individual might well allow one to separate the factors that affect participation in criminal activity from those that affect its timing and duration. We believe that the models we develop here would be useful in doing this.

Models Based on the Exponential Distribution

In this section, we consider models in which the time until recidivism (conditional on eventual recidivism) follows an exponential distribution. However, both the mean of this distribution and the probability of eventual recidivism are allowed to vary among individuals, because individual characteristics are entered as explanatory variables into both of these parts of the model.

The exponential model is an interesting one to consider because it has a potentially important feature, a constant hazard rate at the individual level. In other words, *for a given individual*, the probability of recidivism in the next unit of time is independent of the time since release. The model assumes no "state dependence." When the release cohort has a decreasing hazard rate, in the exponential model, this is entirely due to heterogeneity of individuals. The failure rate of the group falls over time only because the surviving group is increasingly composed of individuals with low failure rates. A decreasing hazard rate caused by heterogeneity might lead to rather different policies than would be reasonable if the hazard rate falls over time (i.e., there is state dependence) at the individual level. If the hazard rate truly falls over time at the individual level, then policies (such as gate money or halfway houses) that help individuals survive in the period immediately after release may be quite effective. However, if the declining hazard rate in the population is due entirely to heterogeneity of individuals, such programs can be expected to have little effect on the rate of recidivism.

Our model is basically the split exponential model discussed in Chapter 5. For individual i, there is an *unobservable* variable F_i that indicates whether or not individual i will eventually return to prison; the variable F_i equals one for individuals who will eventually fail and zero for individuals who will never fail. The probability of eventual failure for individual i will be denoted δ_i, so that:

$$P(F_i = 1) = \delta_i. \tag{7.1}$$

We allow this probability to differ among individuals (different values of i). As in Chapter 6, let $\mathbf{X}_i$ be a (row) vector of individual characteristics (explanatory variables). Also, let α be the corresponding vector of parameters. Then we assume a logit model for eventual recidivism:

$$\delta_i = 1/[1 + e^{\mathbf{X}_i\alpha}]. \tag{7.2}$$

The second feature of the model is that, for individuals for whom $F_i = 1$, the distribution of time until recidivism is exponential, with parameter (hazard rate) θ_i. That is:

$$g(t|F_i = 1) = \theta_i \, e^{-\theta_i t}. \tag{7.3}$$

Furthermore, we assume that:

$$\ln \theta_i = -\mathbf{X}_i \boldsymbol{\beta}, \tag{7.4}$$

which implies that the mean time until recidivism for individual i (conditional on $F_i = 1$) is:

$$1/\theta_i = e^{\mathbf{X}_i \boldsymbol{\beta}}. \tag{7.5}$$

The way in which we have parameterized the model implies that a positive coefficient (in either $\boldsymbol{\alpha}$ or $\boldsymbol{\beta}$) indicates that the corresponding variable has a positive influence on time until recidivism. Specifically, a positive element of $\boldsymbol{\alpha}$ indicates that an increase in the corresponding element of $\mathbf{X}_i$ makes it less likely that the individual will eventually return to prison. Similarly, a positive element of $\boldsymbol{\beta}$ indicates that an increase in the corresponding element of $\mathbf{X}_i$ increases the mean time until recidivism. We note that this is the opposite of the case for the proportional hazards model of the last chapter, in which a positive coefficient indicated a positive effect on the failure rate and thus a negative effect on time until recidivism. We therefore should expect (or hope) that most or all variables will have coefficients with signs that are *opposite* to those in the proportional hazards model. Such a result would indicate a heartening consistency in our results. (Fortunately, we do indeed find this to be the case.)

To write the likelihood function, we follow the notation of Chapter 5 and define the observable variable R_i, which equals one if individual i returned to prison before the end of the follow-up period and equals zero otherwise. We then have:

$$\ln L = \sum_{i=1}^{N} \{R_i \, [\ln \delta_i + \ln \theta_i - \theta_i t_i] + (1 - R_i) \ln [1 - \delta_i + \delta_i \, e^{-\theta_i t_i}]\}, \tag{7.6}$$

where δ_i and θ_i are as defined earlier, and where t_i is the failure time if R_i equals one and the length of the follow-up period if R_i equals zero.

Having presented the model in its most general form, we now consider some special cases. First, we consider the nonsplit model that corresponds to setting $\delta_i = 1$ above. Under this model, we assume that everyone will eventually return to prison. The distribution of time until recidivism is exponential for each individual, but the mean time until recidivism varies among individuals. We will refer to this model as the *exponential model*. We do not expect this model to be very satisfactory for our application, but we include it because it is a model commonly considered in the failure-time literature; for example, see Kalbfleisch and Prentice (1980, p.31), Lawless (1982, section 6.3), and Cox and Oates (1984, section 6.2). The exponential model was applied previously to the analysis of time until recidivism by Witte and Schmidt (1977).

Second, we consider the split model in which the probability of eventual recidivism is the same for each individual, though the mean time until recidivism still varies among individuals. This corresponds to replacing δ_i as defined in Equation 7.2 with the single parameter δ. We will refer to this model as the *split exponential model.*

Third, we consider the model in which the mean time until recidivism (for the eventual recidivists) is the same for each individual, but the probability of eventual recidivism varies among individuals. This corresponds to replacing δ_i as defined in Equation 7.4 with the single parameter θ. We will refer to this model as the *logit exponential model*, whose name emphasizes the assumption of a logit model for eventual recidivism.

Finally, the model in its most general form (with both the probability of eventual recidivism and the mean time until recidivism depending on individual characteristics) will be referred to as the *logit/individual exponential model.* This model obviously includes the other three models as testable special cases. It is models of this final type that we believe may be the most useful in research on criminal careers.

Results for Exponential Models

In this section, we report our results for the exponential models defined in the last section. We begin with a specification which includes all 15 explanatory variables that were used in the proportional hazards model of Chapter 6: TSERVD, AGE, PRIORS, WHITE, FELON, ALCHY, JUNKY, PROPTY, PERSON, MALE, RULE, MARRIED, SCHOOL, WORKREL, and SUPER. It also includes a constant term, denoted CNST, that was not included in the proportional hazards model (being subsumed into the baseline hazard rate). Our parameter estimates for the exponential model with this specification are given in Tables 7.1 and 7.2 (for the 1978 and 1980 analysis samples, respectively), under the heading Original Specification.

The results are strikingly similar to our previous results for the proportional hazards model. (Compare Tables 7.1 and 7.2 to Tables 6.1 and 6.2, remembering that the signs of the coefficients should be opposite, as they are.) In particular, the *same* variables have coefficients that are insignificantly different from zero (at the 5% level, as indicated by the asymptotic t ratio) in the proportional hazards model as in the exponential model: RULE, SCHOOL, WORKREL, PERSON, and SUPER for both years, as well as MARRIED for 1978 and FELON for 1980. For each year, the six coefficients that are individually insignificant, as judged by their

TABLE 7.1. Exponential model, 1978 analysis sample.

	Final specification		Original specification	
Variable	Coefficient	t ratio	Coefficient	t ratio
TSERVD/100	−1.49950	−9.07	−1.280100	−6.69
AGE/1,000	3.79300	7.61	3.659600	6.97
PRIORS/10	−.93918	−7.14	−.875150	−6.43
WHITE	.48404	5.58	.487310	5.57
FELON	.59866	4.28	.628550	3.81
ALCHY	−.44587	−4.30	−.461060	−4.42
JUNKY	−.33437	−3.48	−.297770	−3.07
PROPTY	−.40312	−2.98	−.407450	−2.56
MALE	−.74729	−3.10	−.724000	−2.99
RULE/100			−3.230100	−1.94
MARRIED			.151480	1.41
SCHOOL/10			.279270	1.41
WORKREL			−.096997	−1.08
PERSON			−.141800	−.59
SUPER			.002920	.03
CNST	4.7421	16.76	4.485100	12.10
ln L	−3,326.5		−3,322.3	

asymptotic t ratios, are also *jointly* insignificant, as judged by the likelihood ratio test of the hypothesis that all six coefficients equal zero. This test statistic equals 8.48 for 1978 and 10.21 for 1980, and these values are less than the conventional critical levels of the chi-squared distribution with six degrees of freedom.[2] We therefore dropped six variables from the specification, for each year, to arrive at the results listed under the heading Final Specification in Tables 7.1 and 7.2.

The results for the final specification of our exponential model are also very similar to the corresponding results for the final specification of the proportional hazards model. For each year, every coefficient has the opposite sign in the exponential model than it had in the proportional hazards model, as it should. The relative magnitudes of the coefficients are very similar across models, as are the sizes of the t ratios. We therefore do not need to discuss these results again in detail; we simply repeat the conclusion given in Chapter 6. The type of individual most likely to return to prison shortly after release is a young, black male who is a drug addict and/or alcoholic, who has a large number of previous incarcerations, and whose previous incarceration was lengthy and for a crime against property.

The likelihood values achieved by the exponential model (final specification) are −3,326.5 and −2,893.7 for 1978 and 1980, respectively, as reported in Table 3.2. These values are much larger than the correspond-

[2] These test statistics are also very similar to those for the proportional hazards model, which were 7.37 and 9.34.

TABLE 7.2. Exponential model, 1980 analysis sample.

Variable	Final specification Coefficient	t ratio	Original specification Coefficient	t ratio
PRIORS/10	−1.05480	−9.54	−1.02070	−9.02
TSERVD/100	−1.18360	−7.90	−1.10460	−6.36
AGE/1,000	4.07170	6.85	4.15270	6.77
ALCHY	−.37459	−3.91	−.36885	−3.81
PROPTY	−.34591	−3.80	−.38113	−3.51
MARRIED	.40576	3.27	.41982	3.34
WHITE	.25316	2.85	.26867	2.99
JUNKY	−.25524	−2.53	−.25677	−2.52
MALE	−.58915	−2.31	−.55294	−2.16
SCHOOL/10			.40934	1.89
WORKREL			−.14636	−1.55
RULE/100			−1.99190	−1.51
FELON			.12741	1.23
SUPER			−.12022	−1.08
PERSON			.11381	.67
CNST	4.4483		4.10010	9.96
ln L	−2,893.7		−2,888.6	

ing values for the exponential model without explanatory variables (Chapter 4), which were −3,430.8 and −3,004.5, respectively. This reflects the joint significance (at any reasonable level) of the coefficients of the variables remaining in our final specification; the chi-squared statistics[3] are over 200. Indeed, the likelihood values achieved by the exponential model with explanatory variables are higher than those achieved by any of the models that did not use explanatory variables.[4] The use of explanatory variables clearly improves the fit of the model to the data. Whether it also improves the predictions of the model for other data sets is less clear, as will be seen later.

We next consider the split exponential model, in which there is a constant probability δ of eventual recidivism, but the mean time until recidivism (for the eventual recidivists) varies among individuals. This corresponds to the previous (exponential) model if $\delta = 1$. For this model (and all our subsequent models), we will consider only the specification that was the final specification for the proportional hazards and exponential models. This seems justified because the question of significance of the various coefficients does not seem to be very sensitive to the choice of model, either in these two models or in the models yet to be considered.

[3] These refer to the likelihood ratio test statistics. The appropriate number of degrees of freedom is nine.

[4] The highest previous likelihood values were −3,340.6 for 1978 (split log-logistic distribution) and −2,955.0 for 1980 (split lognormal distribution). See Table 3.2 for details.

Our results for this model are given in Table 7.3. The coefficients and t ratios reported there are all rather similar to those for the exponential model, as given in Tables 7.1 and 7.2. The splitting parameter δ is estimated to be .58 for 1978 and .72 for 1980. These values are noticeably (and significantly) less than one. Thus restricting δ to equal one, as we did in the previous model, is inappropriate. Furthermore, note that the estimates of the splitting parameter are considerably larger than the values found for the splitting parameter in Chapter 5, for models that did not include explanatory variables. Adding heterogeneity to the model causes the hazard rate to decrease (or, more generally, to decrease faster than it would without heterogeneity), and this decrease in the hazard rate apparently substitutes for the decrease in the hazard rate that would be implied by a smaller fraction of eventual recidivists. The ultimate recidivism rates given by this model, though in the range considered plausible, seem a little high.

The likelihood values achieved by the split exponential model are −3,285.0 and −2,882.0 for 1978 and 1980, respectively, as reported in Table 3.2. These are the highest likelihood values found so far, indicating that this is the best-fitting model yet considered.

The third model we consider is the logit exponential model, in which the probability of eventual recidivism varies among individuals according to a logit model, but the distribution of time until recidivism (for the eventual recidivists) is exponential and depends on the single parameter θ. The results for this model are given in Table 7.4. In terms of coefficients and t ratios, the results are rather similar to those for the models previously considered, though the t ratios tend to be a little larger for this model, at least for 1980. The likelihood values are −3,272.7 and −2,872.2 for 1978 and 1980, respectively, and are higher than those for the previous models. (see Table 3.2.) The fact that the likelihood values are higher for the logit

TABLE 7.3. Split exponential model.

1978 Analysis sample			1980 Analysis sample		
Variable	Coefficient	t ratio	Variable	Coefficient	t ratio
TSERVD/100	−1.67180	−7.87	PRIORS/10	−1.02660	−12.08
AGE/1,000	3.71810	7.98	TSERVD/100	−1.46480	−7.10
PRIORS/10	−1.01760	−9.85	AGE/1,000	4.27540	6.89
WHITE	.48441	4.48	ALCHY	−.44112	−3.76
FELON	.82091	4.48	PROPTY	−.40793	−3.83
ALCHY	−.59707	−4.61	MARRIED	.46932	3.48
JUNKY	−.46267	−3.83	WHITE	.25871	2.49
PROPTY	−.67510	−4.09	JUNKY	−.26876	−2.19
MALE	−.85878	−3.32	MALE	−.65693	−2.41
CNST	4.11190	13.82	CNST	4.05770	11.57
δ	.57883	10.63	δ	.71925	19.85
ln L	−3,285.0		ln L	−2,882.0	

TABLE 7.4. Logit exponential model.

1978 Analysis sample			1980 Analysis sample		
Variable	Coefficient	t ratio	Variable	Coefficient	t ratio
TSERVD/100	−2.38090	−9.72	PRIORS/10	−2.78220	−17.52
AGE/1,000	4.17790	7.51	TSERVD/100	−2.15930	−10.55
PRIORS/10	−1.64120	−8.94	AGE/1,000	6.21540	7.71
WHITE	.62033	5.58	ALCHY	−.50428	−3.92
FELON	.87146	5.26	PROPTY	−.51723	−4.14
ALCHY	−.57388	−4.28	MARRIED	.48333	3.00
JUNKY	−.41555	−3.35	WHITE	.44805	3.67
PROPTY	−.50459	−3.21	JUNKY	−.38669	−2.84
MALE	−.85275	−3.43	MALE	−.67600	−2.05
CNST	.18906	.63	CNST	−.29131	−.72
θ	.03184	1604.00	θ	.03261	1345.00
ln L	−3,272.7		ln L	−2,872.7	

exponential model than for the split exponential model indicates that it is more valuable, in terms of fit, to allow the probability of eventual recidivism to vary among individuals than it is to allow the distribution of time until recidivism (for the eventual recidivists) to vary among individuals.

The last model we consider in this section is the logit/individual exponential model, in which both the probability of eventual recidivism and the conditional distribution of time until recidivism are allowed to depend on explanatory variables. The results for this model are given in Tables 7.5 and 7.6. The likelihood values achieved are −3,255.4 and −2,864.8 for 1978 and 1980, respectively, as reported in Table 3.2. These are higher than the corresponding values for the models previously considered in this section, as they must be (in light of the fact that this model includes those models as special cases). The increases in the values of the likelihood are statistically significant, in the sense that the restrictions that would reduce this model to the previous models are jointly rejected by the likelihood ratio test. Thus we are justified in saying that this model represents an improvement, in terms of fit, over the other models of this section.

The coefficient estimates for this model are a little harder to discuss than for our other models, but broadly speaking, they lead to more or less the same statements about the effects of individual characteristics on time until recidivism. Only a few variables (TSERVD in both years and PRIORS in 1980) have coefficients that are significantly different from zero both in the logit model for eventual recidivism and in the exponential model of time until recidivism. Most of the other variables have coefficients that are significantly different from zero in one of these models but not the other, and a few variables have coefficients that are insignificantly different from zero in both places. It is interesting that only prior record significantly

TABLE 7.5. Logit/individual exponential model, 1978 analysis sample.

	Equation for P (never fail)		Equation for duration, given eventual failure	
Variable	Coefficient	t ratio	Coefficient	t ratio
TSERVD/100	−1.31050	−3.78	−1.444100	−4.75
AGE/1,000	3.77540	4.34	1.422900	1.56
PRIORS/10	−1.98680	−4.91	.039529	.20
WHITE	.74094	4.67	−.131450	−.82
FELON	.35430	1.30	.791840	3.39
ALCHY	−.46571	−2.55	−.249990	−1.48
JUNKY	−.37821	−2.23	−.114890	−.72
PROPTY	−.11487	−.46	−.675990	−3.71
MALE	−.93485	−2.67	.137310	.25
CNST	.12416	.28	3.331900	5.29
	$\ln L = -3{,}255.4$			

TABLE 7.6. Logit/individual exponential model, 1980 analysis sample.

	Equation for P (never fail)		Equation for duration, given eventual failure	
Variable	Coefficient	t ratio	Coefficient	t ratio
PRIORS/10	−2.122600	−4.54	−.478220	−2.19
TSERVD/100	−1.227800	−3.43	−.821400	−2.65
AGE/1,000	4.936100	3.14	1.774400	1.39
ALCHY	−.294810	−1.20	−.266630	−1.43
PROPTY	−.091146	−.36	−.518330	−2.78
MARRIED	.476670	1.55	.066481	.23
WHITE	.845740	3.07	−.359220	−1.87
JUNKY	−.534940	−1.89	.056739	.30
MALE	−1.013900	−2.01	.277060	.52
CNST	−.487320	−.72	3.502400	5.54
	$\ln L = -2{,}864.8$			

affects duration, whereas some personal characteristics (age, race, sex, and addiction) as well as prior record affect the probability of eventual recidivism.

We are asking a lot of our data when we attempt to separate out influences on the probability of recidivism from influences on the timing of recidivism. For example, it is clear from our previous models that ALCHY has a negative effect on survival; at any time after release from the sample sentence, alcoholics are more likely to return to prison than nonalcoholics. This is reflected in a significant negative coefficient of ALCHY in all of our previous models. However, for the present model and the 1980 data set, the coefficient of ALCHY is negative but insignificant in both equations. The appropriate inference is that we simply cannot tell whether the negative effect of ALCHY on recidivism is due to its increasing the chance of eventual recidivism or to its decreasing the time until recidivism for those individuals who will fail eventually.

When a variable has a coefficient that is significant in one equation but not the other, the model indicates that the variable affects one aspect of recidivism but not the other. For example, for both the 1978 and the 1980 samples, we have the result that AGE, MALE, and JUNKY affect the probability of eventual recidivism but not the timing of recidivism for those who will fail eventually. On the other hand, PROPTY affects the timing of recidivism for the eventual recidivists but not the probability of eventual recidivism. These are interesting results. However, given that ours is the first rigorous attempt at such a separation of effects, we believe that these results should be viewed as only suggestive until they are replicated in other studies. (A good reason for this word of caution is that not all of these results are robust enough to withstand a change in distributional assumptions, as we will see shortly.)

It is interesting that age and sex seem to affect the probability of recidivism but not its timing. The Panel on Research on Criminal Careers has concluded that these demographic variables would affect the termination rate but not the frequency of offending. Our results support this conclusion.

Those coefficients that are significantly different from zero are always of the same sign as those in our previous models; in that (strong) sense, our results from this model are in broad accordance with the results previously discussed. The nearest thing to an exception to this rule is the negative coefficient of WHITE in the duration equation for 1980, whose significance level is nearly 5%. As noted earlier, there is some instability in previous results on the effect of race on criminality; therefore, this negative coefficient is probably not too surprising.

Predictions From Exponential Models

In this section, we discuss the predictions of recidivism for the 1978 and 1980 validation samples that are implied by our models based on the exponential distribution. See Table 3.2 for a summary. Basically, we conclude that none of our exponential models with explanatory variables predicts very well.

Consider first the results for the exponential model with explanatory variables, the parameter estimates for which were given in Tables 7.1 and 7.2. The predictions of recidivism for the 1978 and 1980 validation samples that we obtain using these models are not very satisfactory. The overall chi-squared statistics are 314.1 and 375.8, and the maximum differences between the predicted and the actual cdf are .066 and .069. These values are barely better than those for the exponential model without explanatory variables (385.7 and 428.0, and .079 and .075; see Table 3.2). They are not nearly as good as the corresponding values for the best of our models without explanatory variables, the split lognormal model (50.6 and 53.9, and .005 and .023; see Table 3.2). The predictions suffer from the same basic problem as did the predictions of most of the models of Chapters 4 and 5: too many recidivists predicted in the first few months after release and for periods long after release, but too few recidivists predicted for the intermediate period. Indeed, the predictions for the exponential model with explanatory variables are discouragingly similar to those of the exponential model without explanatory variables. Our addition of heterogeneity to the model causes the hazard rate to fall, but *not fast enough* to yield accurate predictions. For example, for 1978 the predicted hazard rate is .008 one month after release, and it has fallen to only .006 after 70 months. Clearly, this is not very different from simply predicting a hazard rate of .007 throughout, as the simple exponential model does (see Table 3.1). Our data obviously require a model that allows for a rapid decrease in the hazard rate, which the exponential model (even with explanatory variables) does not. In other words, it appears that it is important to allow for true state dependence as well as heterogeneity.

We next consider the predictions of the split exponential model with explanatory variables, for which the parameter estimates were given in Table 7.3. These are also rather discouragingly poor. The reason is that although the hazard rate falls more rapidly than in the (not split) exponential model, it still falls too slowly to predict accurately.

The overall chi-squared statistics are 161.7 and 266.5 for 1978 and 1980, respectively, and the maximum differences between the actual and the predicted cdf are .035 and .053. (See Table 3.2.) These values are better than for the exponential model, but they are not as good as those for the best of our models without explanatory variables. Indeed, they are worse than the corresponding values for the split exponential model without explanatory variables (115.2 and 174.2, and .024 and .028; see Table 3.2). Even though the coefficients of our explanatory variables are very significantly different from zero, the inclusion of these variables actually reduces the accuracy of the models' predictions. This somewhat surprising result is presumably a reflection of the inadequacy of the exponential distribution in this application.

Table 3.2 also summarizes results for the predictions of recidivism in the 1978 and 1980 validation samples implied by our logit exponential model, the parameter estimates for which were given in Table 7.4. These predictions are better than for our last two models, but they are still not very good. This can be seen from the overall chi-squared statistics of 115.2 and 215.5, and the maximum differences between actual and predicted cdf values of .025 and .042; though an improvement over the corresponding values for the last two models, these are still much larger than for the best models without explanatory variables. Interestingly, the introduction of a logit model for the splitting parameter (so that different individuals have different probabilities of eventual recidivism) does succeed in making the hazard rate fall fast enough to fit the tail of the distribution satisfactorily.

(For example, the predicted hazard rate for 1978 now falls from .014 to .002 over the 70 months for which we make predictions.) The remaining problem with the logit exponential model, which is intrinsic to the choice of the exponential distribution, is that it can not have an increasing hazard rate, whereas the hazard rate in our data does indeed increase for a few months after release; thus the model predicts poorly for the early period after release.

Finally, we consider our predictions for the logit/individual exponential model, for which the parameter estimates were given in Tables 7.5 and 7.6. These predictions are rather similar to those of the logit exponential model, as discussed in the last paragraph. They are a little worse for 1978 and a little better for 1980. (The overall chi-squared statistics are 120.4 and 181.1, and the maximum differences between the predicted and the actual cdf are .027 and .031. See Table 3.2.) The primary problem is again the overprediction of recidivism in the early period after release.

An overall evaluation of the predictions from our exponential models with explanatory variables is straightforward: they are unsatisfactory. The exponential distribution is a simple one to assume, and the models based on it seemed to yield reasonable estimates of the effects of individual characteristics on time until recidivism. However, at least for our data, it is of little use for prediction.

Models Based on the Lognormal Distribution

In this section, we will define models in which time until recidivism (conditional on eventual recidivism) follows a lognormal distribution. These models will be very similar to the models based on the exponential distribution, in that both the mean of the distribution and the probability of eventual recidivism will be allowed to depend on explanatory variables. The only difference is the assumption of the lognormal distribution rather than the exponential.

Specifically, we again assume that the probability of eventual recidivism for individual i, represented by δ_i, is given by the logit model of Equation 7.2. However, we assume that the distribution of time until recidivism (given eventual recidivism) is lognormal, so that the distribution of $\ln t_i$ is normal, with mean μ_i and variance σ^2. The mean of this distribution[5] is assumed to depend on individual characteristics $\mathbf{X}_i$:

$$\mu_i = \mathbf{X}_i \boldsymbol{\beta}. \tag{7.7}$$

[5] Note that μ_i is the mean of the distribution of $\ln t_i$. The mean of the distribution of t_i is:

$$E(t_i) = e^{\mu_i + \sigma^2/2}.$$

Note that, as in the exponential case, the way in which we have parameterized the model implies that a positive coefficient (in either $\boldsymbol{\alpha}$ of Equation 7.2 or $\boldsymbol{\beta}$ of Equation 7.7) indicates that the corresponding variable has a positive influence on time until recidivism (i.e., it makes recidivism either less likely or longer in coming, or both).

To write the likelihood function, we again use the indicator variable R_i, which equals one if individual i returned to prison during the follow-up period. We then have the likelihood:

$$\ln L = \sum_{i=1}^{N} \{R_i\,[\ln \delta_i - 0.5 \ln (2\pi) - 0.5 \ln \sigma^2 - (\ln t_i - \mathbf{X}_i\boldsymbol{\beta})^2/2\sigma^2] + (1 - R_i) \ln P_i\}, \tag{7.8}$$

where

$$P_i = 1 - \delta_i + \delta_i\, \Phi\, [(\mathbf{X}_i\boldsymbol{\beta} - \ln t_i)/\sigma], \tag{7.9}$$

and where Φ is the standard normal cdf.

As with the models based on the exponential distribution, we can now define special cases of this general model. First, the model in which $\delta_i = 1$ (so that everyone eventually would return to prison), but whose mean time until recidivism depends on individual characteristics, will be called the *lognormal model* (with explanatory variables). This model has been considered by Kalbfleisch and Prentice (1980, section 3.6) and Lawless (1982, section 6.5), among others. Witte and Schmidt (1977) have used a very similar model to analyze recidivism.[6] It is not a split model. Second, the model in which δ_i is replaced by a single parameter δ will be referred to as the *split lognormal model* (with explanatory variables). In this model, the probability of eventual recidivism is a constant, though not necessarily equal to one, but the mean of the distribution of time until recidivism varies among individuals. Third, the model in which μ_i is replaced by a single parameter μ will be called the *logit lognormal model*. In this model, the probability of eventual recidivism varies among individuals, but the distribution of time until recidivism (for the eventual recidivists) does not depend on individual characteristics. Finally, the general model as presented earlier will be called the *logit/individual lognormal model*. In this model, both the probability of eventual recidivism and the distribution of time until recidivism vary among individuals. All of these names are consistent with the names for the corresponding exponential models defined earlier in this chapter.

---

[6] The model used by Witte and Schmidt is the model of Amemiya and Boskin (1974). It differs from the lognormal model considered here in the way in which explanatory variables are entered. In particular, it assumes that the mean of time until recidivism (instead of the mean of the logarithm of time until recidivism) is linear in the explanatory variables.

Results for Lognormal Models

In this section, we will present the parameter estimates for our various models based on the lognormal distribution. These estimates are all very similar to those previously presented for the exponential distribution, so they do not require much additional discussion.

We begin with the lognormal model with no splitting parameter, for which the results are given in Table 7.7. The results are all very similar to those for the exponential model (Tables 7.1 and 7.2), which in turn were very similar to those based on the proportional hazards model. Every coefficient is of the same sign as in the exponential model, and the t ratios are also similar in magnitude across models. Once again, the results indicate that the type of individual most prone to early recidivism is a young, black male who is a drug addict and/or alcoholic, who has a large number of previous incarcerations, and whose previous incarceration was lengthy and for a crime against property. Incidentally, the likelihood values achieved were −3,273.0 for 1978 and −2,868.7 for 1980. These are higher than the values for the corresponding exponential model, indicating (unsurprisingly) that the lognormal distribution provides a better fit to the data.

Table 7.8 gives the parameter estimates for the split lognormal model, in which the splitting parameter is a constant, but the mean of the lognormal distribution varies among individuals. Once again, the parameter estimates tell the same story, in terms of the signs of the coefficients and their levels of significance. The splitting parameter is estimated as .71 for 1978 and .94 for 1980. These values are even higher than the values for the split exponential model (.58 and .72, respectively, as reported earlier in this chapter); given the previous results from the literature reviewed in Chapter 5, the splitting parameter for 1980 certainly seems too high. That the

TABLE 7.7. Lognormal model.

1978 Analysis sample			1980 Analysis sample		
Variable	Coefficient	t ratio	Variable	Coefficient	t ratio
TSERVD/100	−2.02030	−6.91	PRIORS/10	−1.41250	−8.78
AGE/1,000	4.00690	7.71	TSERVD/100	−1.35420	−6.21
PRIORS/10	−1.37920	−7.35	AGE/1,000	4.29730	6.79
WHITE	.54160	4.58	ALCHY	−.41234	−3.36
FELON	.88495	4.45	PROPTY	−.38876	−3.52
ALCHY	−.59977	−4.26	MARRIED	.44150	3.29
JUNKY	−.35748	−2.60	WHITE	.27456	2.59
PROPTY	−.59665	−3.13	JUNKY	−.29357	−2.25
MALE	−.85155	−3.17	MALE	−.56707	−2.31
CNST	4.70110	15.53	CNST	4.19530	12.86
σ	1.81830	25.52	σ	1.63920	25.61
ln L	−3,273.0		ln L	−2,868.7	

TABLE 7.8. Split lognormal model.

1978 Analysis sample			1980 Analysis sample		
Variable	Coefficient	t ratio	Variable	Coefficient	t ratio
TSERVD/100	−1.97500	−5.96	PRIORS/10	−1.41260	−8.69
AGE/1,000	3.57210	7.48	TSERVD/100	−1.37100	−5.81
PRIORS/10	−1.45510	−6.66	AGE/1,000	4.25640	6.75
WHITE	.48400	4.10	ALCHY	−.41245	−3.32
FELON	.94958	4.73	PROPTY	−.39094	−3.52
ALCHY	−.61275	−4.21	MARRIED	.44381	3.31
JUNKY	−.31317	−2.18	WHITE	.27127	2.55
PROPTY	−.66631	−3.55	JUNKY	−.28995	−2.19
MALE	−.79656	−3.14	MALE	−.56073	−2.30
CNST	4.08280	13.33	CNST	4.08250	11.00
δ	.70852	17.27	δ	.93838	30.86
σ	1.49010	19.00	σ	1.58810	16.61
ln L	−3,265.1		ln L	−2,868.5	

splitting parameters are larger in the lognormal model than in the exponential model is not surprising, however, because the hazard rate for the lognormal distribution falls fairly rapidly past the first few months. Therefore, there is less need for a small value of the splitting parameter to generate a hazard rate that decreases rapidly enough. The likelihood values achieved are −3,265.1 and −2,868.5 for 1978 and 1980, respectively, which again are larger than those for the corresponding split exponential model.

We next consider the logit lognormal model, in which the splitting parameter varies among individuals, but the mean of the lognormal distribution does not. The parameter estimates for this model are given in Table 7.9. Once again the coefficient estimates and t ratios are more or less the same as before. The likelihood values achieved are −3,256.5 and −2,853.1, which are noticeably higher than for the corresponding logit exponential model. Indeed, this is the highest likelihood value yet achieved for the 1980 data. (See Table 3.2.) For the 1978 data the likelihood value is only slightly smaller than the value for the logit/individual exponential model (which contains eight more parameters). Once again, the lognormal distribution fits our data better than the exponential. The likelihood values are also higher than for the split lognormal model, which contains the same number of parameters. This indicates that, given the choice, it is better to parameterize the probability of eventual recidivism than to parameterize the time until recidivism for the eventual recidivists.

Finally, we consider the logit/individual lognormal model, in which both the probability of eventual recidivism and the distribution of time until recidivism vary according to individual characteristics. These parameter estimates are given in Tables 7.10 and 7.11. They are somewhat more complicated to discuss than the results from our other models, in part because there are simply more parameters, and some of them turn out to be statistically insignificant. However, every coefficient that is significantly

TABLE 7.9. Logit lognormal model.

1978 Analysis sample			1980 Analysis sample		
Variable	Coefficient	t ratio	Variable	Coefficient	t ratio
TSERVD/100	−2.871300	−5.03	PRIORS/10	−3.10870	−6.02
AGE/1,000	4.342400	6.74	TSERVD/100	−2.31500	−4.94
PRIORS/10	−1.985700	−5.26	AGE/1,000	6.43330	6.61
WHITE	.665090	4.79	ALCHY	−.53482	−2.96
FELON	1.004300	4.01	PROPTY	−.55622	−3.39
ALCHY	−.634190	−3.60	MARRIED	.51572	2.69
JUNKY	−.441040	−2.73	WHITE	.47812	3.07
PROPTY	−.558410	−2.35	JUNKY	−.41747	−2.08
MALE	−.882520	−2.96	MALE	−.69187	−1.99
CNST	.067918	.19	CNST	−.40125	−.86
μ	3.215900	43.49	μ	3.08880	43.13
σ	1.200100	23.41	σ	1.17130	22.05
ln L	−3,256.5		ln L	−2,853.082	

TABLE 7.10. Logit/individual lognormal model, 1978 analysis sample.

	Equation for P (never fail)		Equation for duration, given eventual failure	
Variable	Coefficient	t ratio	Coefficient	t ratio
TSERVD/100	−1.584100	−4.63	−1.153200	−3.89
AGE/1,000	3.765300	5.12	1.249800	2.08
PRIORS/10	−1.154300	−4.71	−.665170	−4.01
WHITE	.648180	4.34	.017090	.13
FELON	.463630	1.71	.689110	3.06
ALCHY	−.442800	−2.49	−.312820	−2.07
JUNKY	−.454550	−2.60	.004483	.03
PROPTY	−.204220	−.79	−.567490	−2.85
MALE	−.881170	−2.27	−.097835	−.17
CNST	−.001198	−.00	3.238100	5.43
	σ = 1.1212			
	ln L = −3,239.3			

different from zero has the expected sign (the same sign as in our previous models), and in that sense, the results are still essentially the same as before.

For 1978, four variables have statistically significant effects on both the probability of eventual recidivism and on the mean time until recidivism: TSERVD, AGE, PRIORS, and ALCHY. Three variables have statistically significant effects on the probability but not the timing of recidivism: WHITE, JUNKY, and MALE. The remaining two variables, FELON and PROPTY, have statistically significant effects on the timing of recidivism but not on the probability of eventual recidivism. These results are reasonably similar to the results (given in Table 7.5) for the logit/individual exponential model; the only difference is that AGE, PRIORS, and

TABLE 7.11. Logit/individual lognormal model, 1980 analysis sample.

	Equation for P (never fail)		Equation for duration, given eventual failure	
Variable	Coefficient	t ratio	Coefficient	t ratio
PRIORS/10	−2.85220	−4.65	−.380600	−1.88
TSERVD/100	−2.19180	−3.64	−.324100	−1.44
AGE/1,000	5.67230	4.64	1.385900	1.65
ALCHY	−.36843	−1.69	−.224240	−1.44
PROPTY	−.45773	−2.14	−.134060	−.92
MARRIED	.34823	1.27	.243090	1.18
WHITE	.55001	2.62	−.064623	−.46
JUNKY	−.36728	−1.50	−.081536	−.52
MALE	−.76866	−1.70	.037874	.10
CNST	−.35587	−.62	2.998200	6.58
	$\sigma = 1.1928$			
	$\ln L = -2{,}846.4$			

ALCHY did not have significant effects on the mean time until recidivism in the exponential case.

For 1980, however, the differences across distributions are more substantial. In the logit/individual lognormal model, no variable has a statistically significant effect on the timing of recidivism, and only five variables (PRIORS, TSERVD, AGE, PROPTY, and WHITE) have statistically significant effects on the probability of recidivism. By comparison, in the logit/individual exponential model (Table 7.6), three variables (PRIORS, TSERVD, and PROPTY) had statistically significant effects on the timing of recidivism. Indeed, with respect to the variable PROPTY, the story reverses exactly when we change distributional assumptions. In the lognormal case, PROPTY affects the probability of eventual recidivism but not its timing, whereas in the exponential case, the opposite is true.

What can we conclude from these results? First, if we are to separate the effects of explanatory variables on the probability of recidivism from their effects on its timing, it obviously matters which distribution is chosen; the results from the logit/individual exponential model are noticeably different from the results from the logit/individual lognormal model. This was not true in the simpler models that had only one type of effect for each explanatory variable. (For example, the proportional hazards model, the exponential model, and the lognormal model all yielded essentially identical statements about the effects of explanatory variables on time until recidivism.) The fact that our results are not robust to distributional assumptions clearly weakens our faith in them, as there is never much assurance that one's distributional assumptions are correct. Second, we found it much easier to find significant determinants of the probability of eventual recidivism than to find significant determinants of the timing of recidivism. The explanatory variables in our data are mostly demographic and criminal history variables. It would be very interesting to see whether this same result would occur in an analysis using data that contain more information on environmental variables.

The likelihood values achieved by the logit/individual lognormal model are −3,239.3 and −2,846.4 for 1978 and 1980, respectively. These are the highest likelihood values we have achieved (or will achieve in this book). However, remember that this model has nine more parameters than the logit lognormal model and contains it as a special case, so some increase in the likelihood value is certain to occur in going to this more general model. A relevant question is whether the increase in the likelihood value is statistically significant, or in other words, whether the restrictions that convert this model into the simpler logit lognormal model are rejected by the likelihood ratio test. The likelihood ratio test statistic is twice the difference in the likelihood values and equals 34.4 for 1978 and 13.4 for 1980. The value for 1978 is significant (at usual confidence levels), but the value for 1980 is not; for 1980, at least, there is no reason to believe that the additional complexity of the logit/individual lognormal model is required.

In Tables 7.12 and 7.13, we give results for a shrunken specification of the logit/individual lognormal model, gotten by deleting from the original specification those variables with coefficients that were insignificantly different from zero at the 10% level. The deleted coefficients were also jointly insignificant at conventional significance levels. Their deletion had little effect on the coefficients of the remaining variables, though it did increase the t ratios somewhat. The point of this shrunken specification, as will become more apparent in the next section, is to see whether the

TABLE 7.12. Logit/individual lognormal model, 1978 analysis sample (reduced specification).

	Equation for P (never fail)		Equation for duration, given eventual failure	
Variable	Coefficient	t ratio	Coefficient	t ratio
TSERVD/100	−1.201800	−3.75	−1.37740	−4.84
AGE/1,000	3.851600	5.10	1.22970	1.96
PRIORS/10	−1.218700	−4.71	−.63562	−3.72
WHITE	.666660	4.81	—	—
FELON	—	—	.92881	5.09
ALCHY	−.473390	−2.61	−.29970	−2.02
JUNKY	−.470900	−2.92	—	—
PROPTY	—	—	−.67825	−3.94
MALE	−.933640	−3.08	—	—
CNST	−.011114	−.03	3.20060	15.14
	$\sigma = 1.1471$			
	$\ln L = -3,240.8$			

TABLE 7.13. Logit/individual lognormal model, 1980 analysis sample (reduced specification).

	Equation for P (never fail)		Equation for duration, given eventual failure	
Variable	Coefficient	t ratio	Coefficient	t ratio
PRIORS/10	−2.90340	−5.04	−.34575	−1.97
TSERVD/100	−2.41620	−4.42	—	—
AGE/1,000	5.75040	5.31	1.19420	2.04
ALCHY	−.54384	−2.90	—	—
PROPTY	−.56888	−3.26	—	—
MARRIED	.53155	2.69	—	—
JUNKY	−.42104	−2.02	—	—
CNST	−.22252	−.45	2.80880	14.39
	$\sigma = 1.1855$			
	$\ln L = -2{,}850.7$			

predictions of the logit/individual lognormal model can be improved by removing statistically insignificant coefficients.

Predictions From Lognormal Models

In this section, we discuss the predictions of recidivism for the 1978 and 1980 validation samples that are implied by our models based on the lognormal distribution. In brief, the predictions from the best of our models with explanatory variables are quite satisfactory, but they are not better than the predictions from our best models without explanatory variables. If one is interested in making predictions only for random samples of releasees, the use of explanatory variables is an unnecessary complication, at least for our data.

We consider first the results for our lognormal model with explanatory variables, whose parameter estimates were given in Table 7.7. This is not a split model, but the mean time until recidivism varies among individuals. The predictions of recidivism for the 1978 and 1980 validation samples are not very satisfactory. The overall chi-squared statistics are 142.5 and 181.9 for 1978 and 1980, respectively, whereas the maximum differences between the actual and the predicted cdf are .034 and .051, respectively. These values are considerably worse (larger) than the corresponding values for our best models, as can be seen in Table 3.2. They are, in fact, comparable to the values for the predictions based on the lognormal model without explanatory variables (142.2 and 172.4, and .037 and .045). The prediction errors follow the pattern of those for most of our inadequate models: overprediction of recidivism at the very first and in the tail, with underprediction of recidivism in between.

We next consider the split lognormal model with explanatory variables.

This is a split model, but the splitting parameter (the probability of eventual recidivism) is a constant. The parameter estimates for this model were given in Table 7.8. The overall chi-squared statistics for the predictions of this model are 110.7 and 173.9 for 1978 and 1980, respectively, and the maximum differences between the predicted and the actual cdf are .030 and .050, respectively. As can be seen in Table 3.2, the predictions are better than those from the (not split) lognormal model, though not much better, especially for 1980. They are much *worse* than the predictions from the split lognormal model without explanatory variables, which was our most satisfactory model not containing explanatory variables. The density of time until recidivism in the 1978 validation sample that is predicted by the split lognormal model is displayed as the dotted line in Figure 7.1. The prediction errors follow the same pattern as just discussed for the lognormal model: overprediction at first and in the tail, with underprediction in between.

The third model we consider is the logit lognormal model. In this model, the probability of eventual recidivism depends on individual characteristics, but the distribution of time until recidivism (for the eventual recidivists) does not. The parameter estimates for this model were given in Table 7.9, and its predictions of recidivism for the 1978 validation sample are given in Table 7.14 and Figure 7.1. The overall chi-squared statistics are 50.8 and 57.1 for 1978 and 1980, respectively, and the maximum differences between the predicted and the actual cdf are .006 and .024, respectively. As can be seen in Table 3.2, these values are the lowest yet encountered (indeed, the lowest we will encounter in this book) for our models with explanatory variables. They are very similar to the corresponding values (50.6 and 53.9, and .005 and .023) for the best of our models without explanatory variables, the split lognormal model of chapter 5. The predictions are quite satisfactory for all lengths of time after release, except for the tendency to underpredict the recidivism rate in the 1980 validation sample, which is common to all of our models. Thus we have succeeded in finding a model whose explanatory variables are significantly related to recidivism and that accurately predicts recidivism in our validation samples. However, we have not succeeded in finding a model that predicts recidivism in our validation samples *more* accurately than our best models without explanatory variables. For visual evidence of this fact, compare the relevant curves from Figures 5.1 and 7.1.

The last model we consider is the logit/individual lognormal model, in which both the probability of eventual recidivism and the timing of recidivism vary among individuals. For the full specification (all variables included in both equations), the parameter estimates were given in Tables 7.10 and 7.11. The overall chi-squared statistics for the predictions of these models are 51.0 and 62.9 for 1978 and 1980, respectively, and the maximum differences between the predicted and the actual cdf are .007 and .028, respectively. These values are quite similar to those just reported for

TABLE 7.14. Predicted versus actual recidivism rates for 1978 validation sample using logit lognormal model fit to 1978 analysis sample.

N	Predicted cdf	cdf	t	Predicted density	Density	t	Predicted hazard	Hazard	t	χ^2	df
0	.000	.000	−.89	.000	.000	−.89	.000	.000	−.89	—	—
1	.004	.005	.67	.004	.005	−.91	.004	.005	.91	0.4	1
2	.013	.010	−1.46	.008	.005	−2.29	.008	.005	−2.29	5.7	2
3	.023	.019	−1.55	.011	.009	−.68	.011	.010	−.69	6.1	3
4	.035	.031	−1.43	.012	.011	−.27	.012	.012	−.29	6.2	4
5	.048	.042	−1.52	.012	.011	−.53	.013	.012	−.55	6.5	5
6	.060	.055	−1.26	.013	.013	.22	.013	.014	.21	6.6	6
7	.073	.069	−.82	.012	.014	.77	.013	.015	.77	7.2	7
8	.085	.082	−.54	.012	.013	.58	.013	.014	.62	7.6	8
9	.097	.094	−.53	.012	.012	−.06	.013	.013	−.01	7.6	9
10	.108	.107	−.28	.011	.013	.66	.012	.014	.73	8.1	10
11	.119	.119	−.09	.011	.012	.55	.012	.013	.63	8.5	11
12	.130	.131	.21	.011	.012	.97	.012	.014	1.09	9.7	12
13	.140	.144	.62	.010	.013	1.41	.011	.015	1.56	12.1	13
14	.149	.151	.30	.010	.008	−1.08	.011	.009	−.94	13.0	14
15	.159	.160	.11	.009	.008	−.68	.011	.010	−.54	13.3	15
16	.168	.171	.53	.009	.012	1.65	.010	.014	1.83	16.6	16
17	.176	.178	.32	.009	.007	−.83	.010	.009	−.67	17.1	17
18	.184	.186	.26	.008	.008	−.23	.010	.009	−.06	17.1	18
19	.192	.193	.16	.008	.007	−.43	.009	.009	−.27	17.1	19
20	.200	.200	.06	.007	.007	−.44	.009	.008	−.28	17.2	20
21	.207	.206	−.13	.007	.006	−.88	.009	.007	−.73	17.8	21
22	.214	.212	−.23	.007	.006	−.48	.008	.008	−.34	17.9	22
23	.220	.218	−.38	.007	.006	−.75	.008	.007	−.62	18.2	23
24	.227	.224	−.31	.006	.007	.33	.008	.009	.47	18.5	24
25	.233	.232	−.17	.006	.007	.75	.008	.009	.89	19.3	25
26	.239	.239	.01	.006	.007	.93	.007	.009	1.09	20.4	26
27	.244	.245	.08	.006	.006	.40	.007	.008	.56	20.8	27
28	.250	.251	.13	.005	.006	.32	.007	.008	.48	21.0	28
29	.255	.258	.34	.005	.007	1.24	.007	.009	1.40	23.0	29
30	.260	.262	.24	.005	.004	−.63	.007	.006	−.49	23.2	30
31	.265	.264	−.10	.005	.002	−2.05	.006	.003	−1.96	27.0	31
32	.270	.267	−.36	.005	.003	−1.68	.006	.004	−1.59	29.6	32
33	.274	.271	−.40	.004	.004	−.23	.006	.006	−.13	29.6	33

34	.278	.276	−.37	.004	.005	.18	.006	.006	.28	29.7	34
35	.283	.280	−.32	.004	.005	.31	.006	.006	.42	29.8	35
36	.287	.284	−.34	.004	.004	−.13	.005	.005	−.02	29.8	36
37	.291	.288	−.26	.004	.005	.57	.005	.006	.68	30.3	37
38	.294	.291	−.36	.004	.003	−.77	.005	.004	−.68	30.8	38
39	.298	.295	−.41	.004	.003	−.37	.005	.005	−.28	30.8	39
40	.301	.298	−.49	.004	.003	−.57	.005	.004	−.48	31.1	40
41	.305	.301	−.47	.003	.004	.15	.005	.005	.24	31.1	41
42	.308	.303	−.63	.003	.002	−1.31	.005	.003	−1.25	32.7	42
43	.311	.307	−.50	.003	.004	1.01	.004	.006	1.09	33.9	43
44	.314	.310	−.57	.003	.003	−.50	.004	.004	−.43	34.1	44
45	.317	.314	−.49	.003	.004	.58	.004	.005	.65	34.5	45
46	.320	.317	−.41	.003	.004	.68	.004	.005	.76	35.1	46
47	.323	.319	−.52	.003	.002	−.91	.004	.003	−.86	35.8	47
48	.326	.323	−.37	.003	.004	1.23	.004	.006	1.31	37.5	48
49	.329	.325	−.42	.003	.002	−.41	.004	.003	−.35	37.6	49
50	.331	.328	−.34	.003	.003	.73	.004	.005	.80	38.3	50
51	.334	.329	−.52	.003	.001	−1.70	.004	.001	−1.66	41.0	51
52	.336	.332	−.50	.002	.003	.19	.004	.004	.24	41.1	52
53	.338	.334	−.59	.002	.002	−.84	.003	.002	−.81	41.8	53
54	.341	.336	−.64	.002	.002	−.40	.003	.003	−.37	41.9	54
55	.343	.337	−.75	.002	.001	−1.10	.003	.002	−1.08	43.1	55
56	.345	.340	−.66	.002	.003	.90	.003	.004	.92	43.9	56
57	.347	.342	−.60	.002	.003	.59	.003	.004	.61	44.3	57
58	.349	.344	−.61	.002	.002	−.13	.003	.003	−.11	44.3	58
59	.351	.346	−.65	.002	.002	−.46	.003	.002	−.45	44.5	59
60	.353	.348	−.61	.002	.002	.42	.003	.003	.43	44.7	60
61	.355	.352	−.45	.002	.003	1.73	.003	.005	1.75	44.7	61
62	.357	.354	−.39	.002	.002	.56	.003	.004	.57	48.1	62
63	.359	.356	−.33	.002	.002	.63	.003	.004	.64	48.5	63
64	.361	.358	−.31	.002	.002	.26	.003	.003	.28	48.6	64
65	.362	.361	−.20	.002	.003	1.20	.003	.004	1.22	50.0	65
66	.364	.363	−.13	.002	.002	.83	.003	.004	.85	50.8	66
67	.366	.365	−.13	.002	.002	.00	.003	.003	.01	—	—
68	.367	.366	−.16	.002	.001	−.39	.002	.002	−.39	50.8	67
69	.369	.367	−.15	.002	.002	.12	.002	.003	−.12	—	—
70	.370	.369	−.17	.002	.001	−.29	.002	.002	−.30	50.8	68

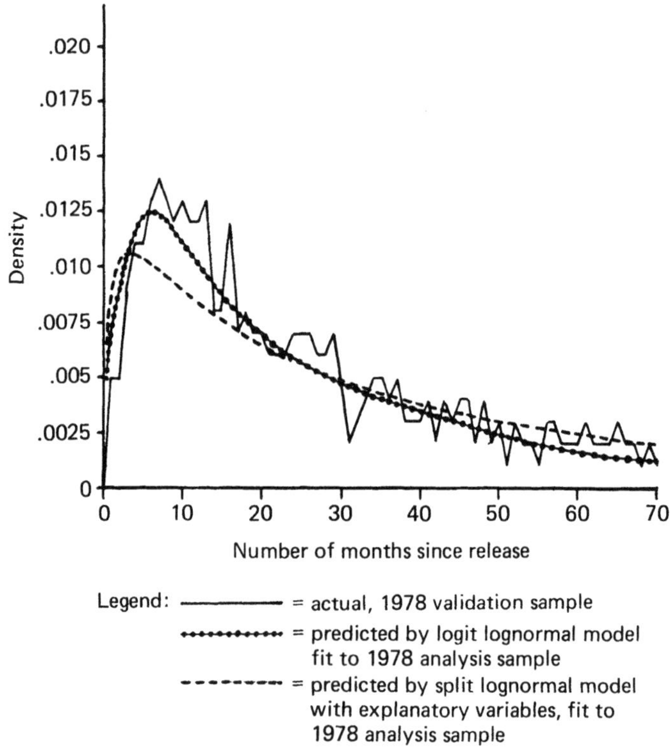

FIGURE 7.1. Predicted versus actual recidivism in the 1978 validation sample: logit lognormal and split lognormal models.

the logit lognormal model, as are the predictions themselves. In terms of the quality of the predictions generated, there is no great loss, but no particular gain, in going from the logit lognormal model to the more complicated logit/individual lognormal model. One possible reason is that not many variables had statistically significant effects on the timing of recidivism in this model, especially for 1980.

In an attempt to improve the predictions of the logit/individual lognormal model, we also considered a shrunken specification, in which some of the variables that had statistically insignificant coefficients were deleted from the model.[7] The parameter estimates for this shrunken specification were given in Tables 7.12 and 7.13. The overall chi-squared statistics for the predictions of these reduced specifications are 51.6 and 60.0 for 1978 and 1980, respectively, and the maximum differences between the predicted and the actual cdf are .013 and .027, respectively. As these sum-

[7] After these variables were deleted, the model was reestimated, so that the coefficients of the remaining variables were changed somewhat.

mary statistics make clear, shrinking the specification of the logit/individual lognormal model does not improve its predictions, which are still slightly inferior to those generated by the logit lognormal model.

A Model Based on the LaGuerre Distribution

We attempted to consider models with explanatory variables that were based on the LaGuerre distribution, but our effort was basically unsuccessful. The model we considered was a logit/individual LaGuerre model, which was similar in spirit to the logit/individual exponential and logit/individual lognormal models described previously. Thus the splitting parameter varied among individuals according to a logit model, exactly as in Equation 7.2. The distribution of time until recidivism (conditional on eventual recidivism) was assumed to follow a second-degree LaGuerre distribution, as given in Chapter 4 (especially Equations 4.9 through 4.11). In this distribution, the parameter α was assumed to vary among individuals, with $\alpha_i = \mathbf{X}_i \boldsymbol{\beta}$.[8]

Though this is an apparently reasonable model, our attempt to maximize its likelihood function encountered serious difficulties. The requirement that the density be positive for every individual failed for almost all parameter values. Accordingly, the likelihood values achieved were only −3,294.5 for 1978 and −2,911.5 for 1980, as can be seen in Table 3.2. These are much lower than the values for the corresponding exponential and lognormal models. The parameter values and t ratios did not make a great deal of sense. Furthermore, the predictions of recidivism that this model generated were very poor. The overall chi-squared statistics were 229.7 and 506.7 for 1978 and 1980, respectively, and the maximum differences between the predicted and the actual cdf were .061 and .085, respectively. These are some of the worst predictions yet encountered, for any model. We therefore gave up on further considerations of the LaGuerre model.

Conclusions

In this chapter, we have estimated parametric statistical models of time until recidivism that have contained individual characteristics as explanatory variables. We have allowed both the probability of eventual recidivism and the distribution of time until recidivism (conditional on eventual

---

[8] Note that the parameter α is as defined in the section of Chapter 4 that discusses the LaGuerre model, and it follows the notation of that section. It is not the same parameter as the parameter α in the notation of this chapter (e.g., Equation 7.2).

recidivism) to depend on such individual characteristics. The probability of eventual recidivism was assumed to follow a logit model. We tried three different distributions (exponential, lognormal, and LaGuerre) for the distribution of time until recidivism, and we obtained reasonable results from two of these distributions (exponential and lognormal).

In some of our models, we allowed only *one* of the two aspects of recidivism (the probability of eventual recidivism and the timing of recidivism for the eventual recidivists) to depend on individual characteristics. For these models, our parameter estimates were entirely straightforward. More significantly, they did not depend much on the model chosen. The results for the exponential models were very similar to those for the lognormal models, and both sets were very similar to the results for the proportional hazards model of Chapter 6. These results indicate that the type of individual most likely to return to prison is a young, black male who is a drug addict and/or alcoholic, who has a large number of previous incarcerations, and whose previous incarceration was lengthy and for a crime against property.

When both the probability of eventual recidivism and the timing of recidivism are allowed to depend on individual characteristics, the parameter estimates are a bit harder to interpret. For most variables, the coefficient in one of the two equations (probability and timing) is statistically insignificant. In some cases, both coefficients are statistically insignificant, even though the variable has a very significant coefficient in our simpler models. Furthermore, these conclusions now change according to the distribution chosen. (For example, for 1980, PROPTY affects the probability of eventual recidivism but not its timing in the lognormal model, but the opposite is true in the exponential model.) Such sensitivity of conclusions to the choice of distribution is unfortunate, as there is never much assurance that we have picked the "correct" distribution. One interpretation of these results is that our data simply are not capable of distinguishing the effects of variables on the probability of eventual recidivism from the effects on its timing. It may be more reasonable to allow only one of these features of recidivism to depend on individual characteristics. In this case, our results clearly indicate that it is more important to allow the probability of eventual recidivism (the splitting parameter) to vary among individuals than it is to allow the mean time until recidivism to vary.

We believe, however, that models allowing both the splitting parameter and the timing of criminal activity to depend on explanatory variables deserve further use and development. In the context of recidivism, such future work may require a richer variety of explanatory variables than we had available in our data. As noted earlier, such models seem potentially quite useful for work seeking to investigate the career criminal paradigm. We would be very interested in seeing this application of our models.

Because a parametric model puts a great deal of structure on the distribution of time until recidivism, the choice of distribution affects the predictions of recidivism to a much larger extent than it affects the parameter estimates. Our lognormal models predict the recidivism rates of the 1978 and 1980 validation samples much better than our exponential models do. (Lognormal models also fit the corresponding estimation samples better.) The best predictions come from the logit lognormal model, in which the probability of eventual recidivism varies among individuals according to a logit model, but the lognormal distribution for the time until recidivism is the same for all eventual recidivists. These predictions are quite satisfactory, except for a tendency to underpredict the rate of recidivism in the 1980 validation sample. This problem is common to all of our models, however, and is simply a reflection of the fact that the recidivism rate is higher in the 1980 validation sample than in the 1980 analysis sample.

However, the predictions for random samples of releasees from our best model with explanatory variables, the logit lognormal model, are no better than the predictions for random samples of releasees from our best model without explanatory variables, the split lognormal model of Chapter 5. Compare Figures 5.1 and 7.1 for visual confirmation of this fact. This is perhaps surprising. When we use a model without explanatory variables, we are considering the marginal distribution of time until recidivism. When we use a model with explanatory variables, we are considering the distribution of time until recidivism *conditional* on these variables. Either distribution can generate satisfactory predictions of recidivism, but the variance of the conditional distribution should be smaller than the variance of the marginal distribution. Therefore, the predictions based on the conditional distribution should, in principle, be more accurate. For example, in a linear regression model, the summary statistic R^2 indicates the fraction of the variance in the dependent variable that is explained by the explanatory variables, so that $1 - R^2$ indicates the variance of the conditional distribution as a fraction of the variance of the marginal distribution. Our models are not linear regression models, but the same sort of statement should hold true. The explanatory variables in our logit lognormal models have the same level of (joint) statistical significance as they would in a linear regression model with an R^2 of .10 for 1978 and .12 for 1980.[9] This clearly indicates that our explanatory variables do not explain a great deal of the variance in time until recidivism, although they do explain about the same proportion of variance as previous studies. (See chapter 1 for a discussion.) Perhaps, then, it is not surprising that our best models with explanatory variables do not predict better (or, in fact, much

[9] The formula is $R^2 = CS/(N - K + CS)$, where CS is the likelihood ratio chi-squared test statistic used to test the statistical significance of the explanatory variables, N is the number of observations, and K is the number of explanatory variables, excluding the constant. We have $CS = 171.0$, $N = 1540$, and $K = 9$ for 1978, and $CS = 203.8$, $N = 1435$, and $K = 9$ for 1980.

differently) than our best models without explanatory variables. After all, we do not have a particularly satisfactory set of explanatory variables, and considerable shrinkage is common in heavily parameterized models, such as those considered in this chapter.

This does not mean that our models with explanatory variables are useless. Even at their current state of development, they have a number of advantages. First, they can be used to rank individuals according to their probabilities of recidivism. (Of course, given the modest fit of the models that generate the rankings, it remains to be seen how useful such rankings would be in predicting individual outcomes.) Second, we can use models with explanatory variables to make predictions for groups that (unlike our validation samples) are not representative of the sample from which the models were estimated. To the extent that the models are accurate, they can at least correct for differences in measured variables between the estimation sample and the group for whom predictions are desired. We will consider individual predictions, as well as predictions for nonrandom subsamples of the release cohort, in the next chapter.

8

Predictions for Nonrandom Samples and for Individuals

Introduction

In previous chapters, we have considered predictions of recidivism for random samples of our release cohorts. Such random samples will differ significantly from the random samples used to estimate our models only by chance. We now turn to the much more difficult task of making predictions for groups that differ systematically from the samples used in estimation. This type of prediction has often been strongly recommended but rarely pursued in practice.[1] We also consider predictions of recidivism at the individual level. Making either of these types of predictions requires a model that includes individual characteristics as explanatory variables. This is obviously the case with individual predictions, as a model that did not include individual characteristics would only predict the same distribution of time until recidivism for every individual. On the other hand, in the case of predictions for groups that are nonrandom samples of the release cohort, the purpose of having individual characteristics in the model is to correct for differences between the group in question and the rest of the cohort. For example, in making predictions of the rate of recidivism of a group of youthful offenders, the model can account for the age of the individuals (assuming that age was a variable used in the model), as well as for differences between the group and the estimation sample in the values of the other relevant explanatory variables.

In this chapter, we consider three specific types of prediction problems. First, we investigate whether models estimated using data on the 1978 release cohort can predict accurately the rate of recidivism in the 1980 cohort. This is the type of cross-cohort prediction carried out by Gottfredson and Gottfredson (1985), who estimated their model using a sample of federal releasees for 1970 and then made predictions for a similar sample of 1972 releasees. In our case, this is more difficult to do because

[1] Gottfredson and Gottfredson (1985) is an exception in this regard.

the recidivism rate in the 1980 data is significantly higher than in the 1978 data. Therefore, models fit to the 1978 data tend to underpredict the rate of recidivism in the 1980 data. However, we are reasonably successful; most of the difference in recidivism rates across the two cohorts is explained by differences in observable characteristics of the releasees. (See Chapter 2 for a discussion of the observable differences between the two cohorts.)

Second, we make predictions for nonrandom subsamples of releasees, such as youthful offenders, alcoholics, felons, and so forth. These predictions unfortunately are not very accurate, and this finding is not encouraging to the use of our models in the evaluation of correctional programs applied to nonrandom groups of releasees. It appears that we have entered the explanatory variables into our models in too simple a manner, and they do not adequately capture the effects of the explanatory variables on time until recidivism. With more work on the ways in which explanatory variables should be entered into the models, there is hope that this pessimistic conclusion can be reversed. For example, our previous work (Schmidt & Witte, 1978, 1984) suggests that predictions for nonrandom groups can be improved if separate models are estimated for different race, sex, and age groups.

Finally, we make predictions for individuals. Each of our models can be used to score individuals, with the higher scores representing a higher probability of recidivism. Our scores do predict recidivism but only with considerable randomness (noise) remaining. The accuracy of prediction at the individual level is probably not high enough for our models to be very useful for implementing a policy of selective incapacitation. However, we are able to predict the criminal activity of individuals more accurately than a number of other recent studies (e.g., Blumstein et al., 1985; Greenwood, 1982). Furthermore, we succeed in keeping both our false positive and false negative rates below 50%. This is a criterion suggested by Farrington (1987) for judging a prediction study to be successful.

Our false positive rate for the 1978 validation sample is 47%, and our false negative rate is 28%. It is clear that we are much better able to predict who will not return to prison than to predict who will; this is presumably to be expected, as most North Carolina prison releasees do not return to prison. Thus it seems to us far more reasonable to use individual predictions from our models to select inmates for more desirable treatment (lower security levels, work and study release, parole) than to select individuals for harsher treatment, such as longer periods of incarceration.

Predictions Across Release Cohorts

In this section, we use our models of time until recidivism, estimated using data from the 1978 release cohort, to make predictions of the rate of recidivism in the 1980 release cohort. More specifically, the models we use are estimated using data on the 1978 analysis sample, as described in Chapters 4 through 7, and we make predictions of recidivism for the 1980 validation sample. The results are summarized in the last two columns of Table 3.2.

It is interesting to see whether we can make such predictions accurately because practical uses of models like ours (for program evaluation or population projections, for example) will typically rely on the accuracy of these predictions. The difficulty and expense of specifying and estimating models of this type make it unreasonable to expect that they should be reestimated every year, and their usefulness will be limited if they can predict accurately only for the cohort on which they were estimated.

The problem that we face at the outset is that the recidivism rate in the 1980 cohort is considerably higher than in the 1978 cohort. As reported and discussed in the section Comparisons of Subsamples (Chapter 2), the recidivism rate after a follow-up of 46 months (the minimum length in the 1980 data) was .324 for 1978 and .359 for 1980. Similar differences exist for other follow-up periods. Thus we can expect our models based on 1978 data to *underpredict* recidivism in the 1980 data. However, there are also significant differences between the 1978 and 1980 cohorts in the individual characteristics that are explanatory variables in our models of Chapters 6 and 7. The basic question then is how much of the difference in the 1978 and 1980 recidivism rates is explained by these differences in individual characteristics. As we shall see, most of the difference is explainable; the best 1978 models that contain explanatory variables predict the 1980 recidivism rate reasonably well.

The differences in recidivism rates between the 1978 analysis sample and the 1980 validation sample are evident in Figure 8.1. Here we consider a nonparametric "model," in which we simply predict the same proportion of recidivists at each point in time for the 1980 validation sample as in the 1978 analysis sample. (This is the same type of prediction as that considered in the section Nonparametric Predictions in Chapter 4.) In Figure 8.1, the solid line represents the actual density of time until recidivism in the 1980 validation sample, and the dashed line represents the predicted density, which is the actual density in the 1978 estimation sample. It is obvious that we underpredict the recidivism rate in the 1980 validation sample, particularly in the first year after release. This is even more evident in a comparison of the cumulative proportions of returns, which are not reported in Figure 8.1. For example, after 12, 24, 36, and 46 months, the values predicted from the 1978 data are .122, .227, .286, and .318, respectively. The values realized in the 1980 data are .171, .274, .338, and .368, respectively.[2] In terms of the month to month number of recidivists,

---

[2] The 46-month predicted and actual recidivism rates of .318 and .368 differ slightly from the values (.324 and .359) given in the previous paragraph. The explanation for this difference is that the values given in the previous paragraph are based on the entire 1978 and 1980 release cohorts, but the values given here are based on the 1978 analysis sample and the 1980 validation sample.

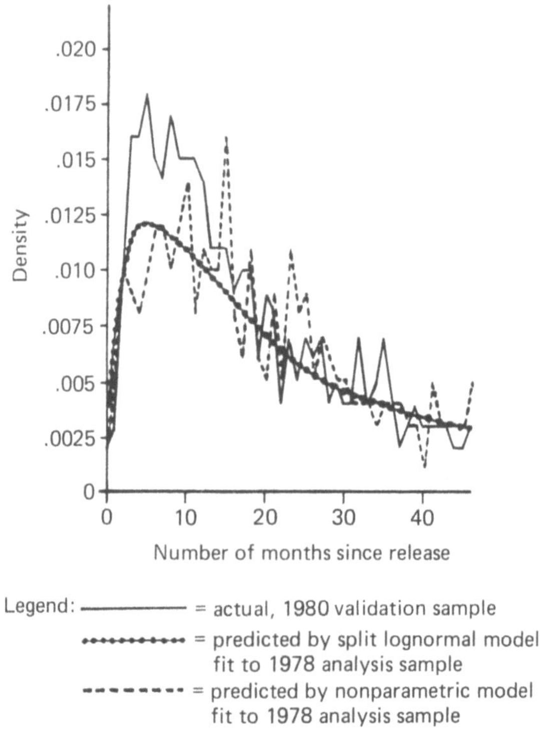

FIGURE 8.1. Predicted versus actual recidivism in the 1980 validation sample: 1978 split lognormal and nonparametric models.

comparisons are less clear because of the large amount of noise in the monthly figures, but the same pattern of underprediction still occurs, at least for the first 18 months after release, as is clear in Figure 8.1.

The overall chi-squared statistic for our nonparametric predictions is 273.1, and the maximum difference between the predicted and the actual cdf is .054. (See the last two entries in the first row of Table 3.2.) These rather large values of the goodness of fit statistics confirm the conclusion of the last paragraph that the 1978 nonparametric model gives unsatisfactory predictions of recidivism for the 1980 cohort. The nonparametric model's underprediction of recidivism is statistically significant, and this remains so even when we correct the chi-squared statistic to reflect the variability of the nonparametric predictions (as described in Chapter 4).

We next turn to our parametric statistical models of time until recidivism. We begin with the simple models of Chapter 4. These are not split models, and they do not contain explanatory variables. The summary statistics for the predictions of the recidivism rate in the 1980 validation sample that are implied by our 1978 models based on the exponential, Weibull, lognormal, log-logistic, and LaGuerre distributions are given again in the last two columns of Table 3.2. It is evident from the summary statistics in Table 3.2 that these models do a very poor job of predicting the recidivism rate in the 1980 validation sample. For example, consider the LaGuerre model, which was the most successful of our models of Chapter 4 and which also gives the most accurate predictions in the present context. The overall chi-squared statistic is 264.6 and the maximum difference between the predicted and the actual cdf is .059. These values are much higher than the corresponding values of 172.1 and .031 for predictions based on the LaGuerre model fit to the 1980 estimation sample. The problem is that the 1978 LaGuerre model *underpredicts* the rate of recidivism in the 1980 data, as was expected.

We next consider our split models of Chapter 5, which do not contain explanatory variables. They are based on the same distributions just considered and are estimated using the 1978 estimation sample. Table 3.2 again gives the summary goodness of fit statistics for these models' predictions for the 1980 validation sample. Though the split models predict better than the simple models previously discussed, the same problem of underprediction occurs. For example, consider the predictions of the split lognormal model, which are displayed as the dotted line in Figure 8.1. Recall that this was our most successful model of Chapter 5 and, indeed, the best model we considered that did not use individual characteristics as explanatory variables. It is also the best model here in the sense that the 1978 split lognormal model predicts the recidivism rate of the 1980 validation sample better than any of the other 1978 split models. However, it still does not predict very well. The overall chi-squared statistic is 126.3 and the maximum difference between the actual and predicted the cdf is .053; these values compare unfavorably with the corresponding values of 53.9 and .023 for predictions based on the 1980 split lognormal model. It is clear from Figure 8.1 that the 1978 split lognormal model significantly underpredicts the recidivism rate in the 1980 validation sample, particularly in the first year after release. The same is true for all of the other split models that do not contain explanatory variables.

We now turn to our models that contain individual characteristics as explanatory variables. Because the recidivism rate in the 1980 cohort exceeds the rate in the 1978 cohort, it is not surprising that the models considered so far should underpredict recidivism in the 1980 data. However, we can hope that the difference in recidivism rates across years can be explained by differences in the values of (observable) individual characteristics in the two cohorts. If so, models that use such individual characteristics as explanatory variables may predict accurately across cohorts.

We first consider the predictions based on the 1978 proportional hazards model. The proportional hazards model was described in Chapter 6. It is a nonparametric model in the sense that, while it makes strong assumptions about the effects of explanatory variables on the hazard rate (i.e., linearity), it places no restrictions on the value of the baseline hazard over time. The 1978 proportional hazards model does not predict the recidivism rate in the 1980 validation sample terribly well. However, it is noteworthy that it predicts about as well as the 1980 proportional hazard model. The overall chi-squared statistic and maximum difference between the predicted and the actual cdf are 197.6 and 0.037 for predictions based on the 1978 proportional hazards model, and these compare favorably with the corresponding values of 232.4 and 0.034 for predictions based on the 1980 proportional hazards model (see Table 3.2). The proportional hazards model underpredicts the rate of recidivism in the 1980 validation sample, and this is true whether it is estimated using the 1978 analysis sample or the 1980 analysis sample. The degree of underprediction is about the same in the two cases. Thus there is evidence that the use of explanatory variables has successfully explained most of the difference in recidivism rates between the two years. What predictive inaccuracy remains appears to be due simply to the use of an inadequate model.

We obtain similiar results for our models based on the exponential distribution. These are the exponential, split exponential, logit exponential, and logit/individual exponential models described in chapter 7; each contains individual characteristics as explanatory variables. These models based on the exponential distribution are not very adequate, and they predict recidivism poorly. However, in three of the four cases, the models estimated using 1978 data predict the recidivism rate in the 1980 validation sample just as well as the corresponding models estimated using 1980 data. The predictive inaccuracy that remains appears to be due to the inadequacy of the exponential model and not to unexplained inter-year variation in the recidivism rate.

Finally, we turn to the predictions implied by our models based on the lognormal distribution. Specifically, we consider the lognormal model, the split lognormal model, the logit lognormal model, the logit/individual lognormal model, and the logit/individual lognormal model with a reduced specification (some statistically insignificant coefficients set to zero). These models are as described in Chapter 7. The summary statistics for these models' predictions of recidivism for the 1980 validation sample are reported in the last five rows of Table 3.2.

In Chapter 7, we reported that the best of these models was the logit lognormal model. It gave the best predictions for both 1978 and 1980. However, its predictions for the 1980 validation sample, but based on the model fit to the 1978 analysis sample, are less satisfactory. For example, the overall chi-squared statistic of 97.6 and the maximum difference between the predicted and the actual cdf of 0.042 are noticeably larger than the corresponding values of 57.1 and 0.024 for predictions based on the 1980 estimates. (See Table 3.2.) Both the 1978 model and the 1980 model underpredict the rate of recidivism in the 1980 validation sample, but the underprediction is worse for the 1978 model.

However, the 1978 logit lognormal model is *not* the 1978 model which best predicts the recidivism rate of the 1980 validation sample. The 1978 logit/individual lognormal model is more successful. Its predictions are still worse than those of the best 1980 model (the 1980 logit lognormal model) but only very marginally worse. This can be seen by comparing Table 8.1, which gives the predictions based on the 1978 logit/individual lognormal model, to Table 8.2, which gives the predictions based on the 1980 logit lognormal model. The predicted densities of time until recidivism based on these two models are also displayed in Figure 8.2. As can easily be seen there is not much difference between them. This similarity is also reflected in the goodness of fit statistics reported in Table 3.2: 57.1 and .024 for the 1980 logit lognormal model, and 61.8 and .032 for the 1978 logit/individual lognormal model.

The logit/individual lognormal model is more flexibly parameterized than the logit lognormal model, because the explanatory variables are allowed to affect the mean time until return for the eventual recidivists as

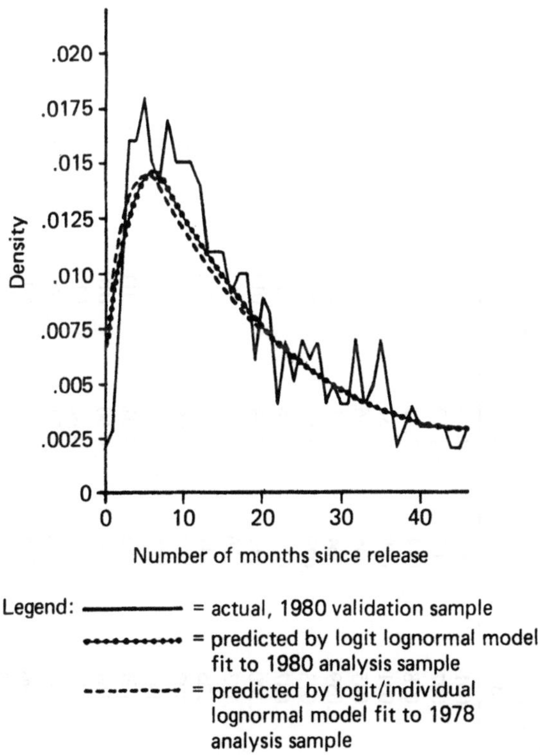

FIGURE 8.2. Predicted versus actual recidivism in the 1980 validation sample: logit lognormal and logit/individual lognormal models.

Table 8.1. Predicted versus actual recidivism rates for 1980 validation sample using logit/individual lognormal model fit to *1978* analysis sample.

N	Predicted cdf	cdf	t	Predicted density	Density	t	Predicted hazard	Hazard	t	χ^2	df
0	.001	.001	1.93	.001	.001	1.93	.001	.001	1.93	—	—
1	.007	.005	−1.79	.006	.003	−2.47	.006	.003	−2.56	3.2	1
2	.018	.014	−1.73	.011	.010	−.76	.011	.010	−.99	4.2	2
3	.031	.030	−.31	.013	.016	1.49	.014	.016	1.14	5.5	3
4	.045	.046	.56	.014	.016	1.40	.015	.017	1.04	6.6	4
5	.059	.064	1.47	.014	.018	1.87	.016	.019	1.56	9.0	5
6	.073	.079	1.64	.014	.015	.65	.016	.016	.37	9.1	6
7	.087	.094	1.66	.014	.014	.33	.015	.016	.08	9.1	7
8	.100	.111	2.49	.013	.017	2.33	.015	.019	2.08	13.4	8
9	.113	.126	2.86	.013	.015	1.33	.015	.017	1.17	14.8	9
10	.125	.141	3.38	.012	.015	1.83	.014	.018	1.69	17.7	10
11	137	.157	3.99	.012	.015	2.21	.014	.018	2.14	22.2	11
12	.148	.171	4.49	.011	.014	2.03	.013	.017	2.00	26.2	12
13	.159	.183	4.51	.011	.011	.48	.013	.014	.52	26.5	13
14	.169	.194	4.60	.010	.011	.68	.012	.014	.72	27.0	14
15	.179	.205	4.82	.010	.011	1.17	.012	.014	1.25	28.6	15
16	.188	.214	4.71	.009	.009	−.08	.011	.011	.01	28.6	16
17	.196	.224	4.80	.009	.010	.71	.011	.012	.82	29.2	17
18	.205	.234	4.98	.008	.010	1.03	.011	.013	1.14	30.5	18
19	.213	.240	4.63	.008	.006	−1.24	.010	.008	−1.13	31.8	19
20	.220	.249	4.86	.008	.009	1.29	.010	.012	1.41	33.8	20

21	.228	.257	4.95	.007	.008	.69	.009	.011	.83	34.5	21
22	.234	.262	4.49	.007	.004	−1.98	.009	.006	−1.87	38.0	22
23	.241	.269	4.51	.007	.007	.29	.009	.009	.40	38.2	23
24	.247	.274	4.31	.006	.005	−.81	.008	.007	−.71	38.7	24
25	.253	.282	4.50	.006	.007	1.17	.008	.010	1.28	40.3	25
26	.259	.287	4.47	.006	.006	.01	.008	.008	.13	40.3	26
27	.265	.294	4.59	.006	.007	.84	.008	.009	.96	41.3	27
28	.270	.298	4.38	.005	.004	−1.03	.007	.006	−.93	42.1	28
29	.275	.303	4.28	.005	.005	−.43	.007	.007	−.32	42.2	29
30	.280	.307	4.11	.005	.004	−.90	.007	.006	−.80	42.9	30
31	.285	.311	4.05	.005	.004	−.29	.007	.006	−.18	42.9	31
32	.289	.318	4.37	.005	.007	2.16	.006	.010	2.29	42.9	32
33	.294	.322	4.32	.004	.004	−.18	.006	.006	−.05	48.1	33
34	.298	.327	4.44	.004	.005	.93	.006	.008	1.07	48.1	34
35	.302	.334	4.80	.004	.007	2.55	.006	.010	2.74	49.3	35
36	.306	.338	4.86	.004	.004	.55	.006	.007	.73	56.8	36
37	.310	.340	4.63	.004	.002	−1.53	.005	.004	−1.40	57.3	37
38	.313	.344	4.57	.004	.003	−.39	.005	.005	−.25	59.3	38
39	.317	.348	4.62	.003	.004	.52	.005	.006	.67	59.8	39
40	.320	.351	4.63	.003	.003	.14	.005	.005	.28	59.9	40
41	.323	.354	4.62	.003	.003	.01	.005	.005	.15	59.9	41
42	.326	.357	4.52	.003	.003	−.68	.005	.004	−.56	60.2	42
43	.329	.360	4.57	.003	.003	.54	.005	.005	.69	60.7	43
44	.332	.362	4.44	.003	.002	−1.02	.004	.003	−.90	61.5	44
45	.335	.365	4.36	.003	.002	−.63	.004	.004	−.51	61.8	45
46	.338	.368	4.35	.003	.003	.06	.004	.004	.19	61.8	46

TABLE 8.2. Predicted versus actual recidivism rates for 1980 validation sample using logit/lognormal model fit to 1980 analysis sample.

N	Predicted cdf	cdf	t	Predicted density	Density	t	Predicted hazard	Hazard	t	χ^2	df
0	.000	.001	4.21	.000	.001	4.21	.000	.001	4.21	—	—
1	.005	.005	−.50	.005	.003	−1.55	.005	.003	−1.54	0.3	1
2	.015	.014	−.47	.010	.010	−.22	.010	.010	−.22	0.3	2
3	.028	.030	.83	.013	.016	1.73	.013	.016	1.72	3.3	3
4	.042	.046	1.51	.014	.016	1.41	.014	.017	1.44	5.3	4
5	.056	.064	2.22	.014	.018	1.74	.015	.019	1.81	8.6	5
6	.071	.079	2.21	.015	.015	.44	.015	.016	.53	8.9	6
7	.085	.094	2.06	.014	.014	.06	.015	.016	.16	8.9	7
8	.099	.111	2.72	.014	.017	1.98	.015	.019	2.10	13.3	8
9	.112	.126	2.93	.013	.015	.97	.015	.017	1.14	14.6	9
10	.125	.141	3.30	.013	.015	1.44	.014	.018	1.63	17.3	10
11	.137	.157	3.77	.012	.015	1.80	.014	.018	2.03	21.4	11
12	.149	.171	4.14	.012	.014	1.61	.013	.017	1.88	24.9	12
13	.160	.183	4.06	.011	.011	.11	.013	.014	.39	25.1	13
14	.171	.194	4.05	.011	.011	.29	.013	.014	.58	25.4	14
15	.181	.205	4.17	.010	.011	.78	.012	.014	1.09	26.6	15
16	.191	.214	3.98	.010	.009	−.44	.012	.011	−.15	26.6	16
17	.200	.224	4.00	.009	.010	.34	.011	.012	.63	27.0	17
18	.209	.234	4.10	.009	.010	.66	.011	.013	.94	27.9	18
19	.217	.240	3.70	.008	.006	−1.54	.010	.008	−1.30	29.6	19
20	.226	.249	3.86	.008	.009	.93	.010	.012	1.19	31.0	20
21	.233	.257	3.90	.008	.008	.35	.010	.011	.62	31.4	21

22	.241	.262	3.40	.007	.004	−2.24	.009	.006	−2.03	35.5	22
23	.248	.269	3.37	.007	.007	−.02	.009	.009	.19	35.6	23
24	.254	.274	3.13	.007	.005	−1.09	.009	.007	−.91	36.4	24
25	.261	.282	3.27	.006	.007	.85	.008	.010	1.05	37.5	25
26	.267	.287	3.20	.006	.006	−.27	.008	.008	−.09	37.5	26
27	.273	.294	3.28	.006	.007	.54	.008	.009	.72	38.0	27
28	.278	.298	3.04	.006	.004	−1.27	.008	.006	−1.14	39.3	28
29	.284	.303	2.91	.005	.005	−.68	.007	.007	−.54	39.6	29
30	.289	.307	2.71	.005	.004	−1.13	.007	.006	−1.01	40.6	30
31	.294	.311	2.61	.005	.004	−.52	.007	.006	−.42	40.8	31
32	.299	.318	2.90	.005	.007	1.86	.007	.010	1.97	44.7	32
33	.303	.322	2.83	.005	.004	−.40	.007	.006	−.31	44.8	33
34	.308	.327	2.92	.004	.005	.68	.006	.008	.78	45.4	34
35	.312	.334	3.25	.004	.007	2.27	.006	.010	2.39	51.1	35
36	.316	.338	3.29	.004	.004	.33	.006	.007	.44	51.3	36
37	.320	.340	3.05	.004	.002	−1.70	.006	.004	−1.62	53.9	37
38	.324	.344	2.96	.004	.003	−.58	.006	.005	−.51	54.2	38
39	.327	.348	2.99	.004	.004	.31	.005	.006	.38	54.3	39
40	.331	.351	2.98	.004	.003	−.05	.005	.005	.00	54.3	40
41	.334	.354	2.95	.003	.003	−.18	.005	.005	−.13	54.4	41
42	.338	.357	2.84	.003	.003	−.84	.005	.004	−.81	55.0	42
43	.341	.360	2.88	.003	.003	.36	.005	.005	.39	55.2	43
44	.344	.362	2.74	.003	.002	−1.16	.005	.003	−1.15	56.5	44
45	.347	.365	2.64	.003	.002	−.78	.005	.004	−.77	57.1	45
46	.350	.368	2.62	.003	.003	−.10	.005	.004	.11	57.1	46

well as the probability of eventual recidivism. This extra flexibility is apparently unnecessary when we use the model to make predictions for the same cohort as was used in estimation, but it is helpful when we make predictions for the 1980 cohort based on the 1978 estimates. The apparent explanation is that this additional flexibility is useful so that differences in explanatory variables can account as fully as possible for differences across years in observed recidivism rates. An important implication is that, if one is estimating models that are to be used to make predictions for future release cohorts, it may be desirable to use models that are more flexibly parameterized than would appear necessary from the data currently available. This conjecture seems worth checking in future work.

The results of this section are easy to summarize. The recidivism rate in the 1980 release cohort exceeds that in the 1978 cohort. Models that do not use individual characteristics as explanatory variables, and which are fit to data on the 1978 cohort, consistently underpredict the rate of recidivism in the 1980 cohort. On the other hand, models that use individual characteristics as explanatory variables typically predict the 1980 recidivism rate equally well when fit to 1978 data as when fit to 1980 data. In particular, the best models fit to the 1978 data predict the 1980 recidivism rate reasonably well; at least, they predict it about as well as the best models fit to the 1980 data. In that sense, differences across cohorts in the values of observable individual characteristics account for virtually all of the observed difference in recidivism rates across cohorts.

Although the primary purpose of this book is methodological, we also wished to provide the North Carolina Department of Correction with models that would allow them to predict the behavior of future release cohorts. We had previously provided the Department with such models in 1978 (Schmidt & Witte, 1978, 1984). These models were based on the lognormal distribution, and they were estimated using data on a cohort of individuals released during the first 6 months of 1975. In this earlier work, we explored alternative distributional assumptions to a much lesser degree than we do here. However, we explored the proper parameterization of the effects of explanatory variables on time until recidivism to a much greater degree. Specifically, instead of stopping after estimating a single set of parameters for our cohort, we proceeded to obtain separate parameter estimates for five different race, age, and sex groups.[3] We found that these group-specific models predicted better than our model for the entire cohort but only for two of the five groups, females and nonblack male adults. For the other three groups (black male adults and both black and nonblack male youths), the general population model predicted better than the group-specific models. Using the group-specific models for females and

[3] The groups are females, nonblack male adults, black male adults, black male youths, and nonblack male youths. See Schmidt and Witte (1978) or Chapter 7 of Schmidt and Witte (1984) for details.

nonblack male adults, and the general population model for all other groups, we were able to improve predictive accuracy markedly.

When we delivered the models described above to the North Carolina Department of Correction in 1978, we advised them to check annually the predictive accuracy of the models by using them to predict the timing of recidivism for random samples of releasees (see Schmidt & Witte, 1978). The Department followed our advice and found that the models continued to predict quite well until the early 1980s.[4] These results are, of course, consistent with our ability to predict recidivism accurately for 1980 releasees by using models estimated with data on 1978 releasees. It would appear that the characteristics of releasees change much more rapidly than their underlying behavior, as reflected in the parameter estimates. Thus it appears that parametric models that explicitly incorporate explanatory variables (models like those of Chapter 7) can be expected to predict the recidivism experience of future release cohorts for some time. This is important because it means that prediction models may not have to be reestimated every year.

Subsample Predictions

In this section, we report the predictions of our best-fitting model, the logit lognormal model, for nonrandom subsamples of the release cohort. We will make predictions for 11 different groups of releasees, including youthful offenders and participants in the North Carolina prisoner work release program. The accuracy of such predictions is another good check of our model's adequacy. The model contains as explanatory variables the individual characteristics that define our subsamples (for example, AGE and WORKREL for the groups mentioned above). If we have adequately captured the effects of these variables on time until recidivism, the model should predict accurately for subsamples of the type we consider and not just for the whole sample.

Another reason for our interest in the accuracy of predictions for subsamples is that this is exactly the kind of prediction that is needed if our models are to be used for program evaluation. We have previously suggested that programs can be evaluated by comparing the actual rate of recidivism in a treatment group with the recidivism rate predicted by an adequate model (Schmidt & Witte, 1979; 1984, chap. 8). In doing this, we are essentially using the entire release cohort as the control group and using the model to control for differences in individual characteristics between the control group and the treatment group. If we know which group is being treated at the time the model is estimated, a more standard

[4] Personal communication from Mr. Ken Parker, Research Division, North Carolina Department of Correction (February 1985).

procedure would be to include one or more variables indicating the treatment in the model and to test their significance. The model then controls for differences in measured characteristics between the treatment and nontreatment group. (This is exactly what is done in the biostatistical literature, where one may use a survival time model to estimate the effect of a drug on the survival of cancer patients, while controlling for concomitant variables such as age and severity of pre-treatment condition. As a typical example, see Prentice [1973], cited by Lawless [1982, p. 273].) However, the identification and estimation of an adequate survival time model is extremely costly and time-consuming, while the use of such a model to make predictions is relatively cheap and simple. The "predicted versus actual" technique that we previously suggested is therefore a potentially cost-effective way to evaluate programs or, at least, to screen programs to see which may be worth the expense of a more rigorous evaluation. However, as treatments are typically applied to groups that are nonrepresentative of the entire release cohort,[5] it is important that the model used is capable of predicting accurately the recidivism rate in nonrepresentative subsamples. This is what we now proceed to check for our logit lognormal model.

We make predictions for 11 different groups of releasees: blacks (WHITE = 0), participants in the work release program (WORKREL = 1), youthful offenders (AGE < 252, i.e., under 21 years of age), older offenders (AGE ⩾ 480, i.e., age greater than or equal to 40 years), alcoholics (ALCHY = 1), users of hard drugs (JUNKY = 1), felons (FELON = 1), females (MALE = 0), property offenders (PROPTY = 1), individuals who have served long sentences (TSERVD > 12 months), and individuals with more than one prior incarceration (PRIORS > 0)[6]. We make these predictions for both 1978 and 1980, and we also use the 1978 model to make predictions for these subsamples of the 1980 validation sample.

Table 8.3 gives the group sizes and summary statistics (the overall chi-squared statistic and the maximum difference between predicted and actual cdf) for these predictions. For the 1978 data,[7] Tables 8.4 through 8.6 give a detailed listing of these predictions for 3 of the 11 groups described above: blacks (Table 8.4), participants in the work release program (Table 8.5), and youthful offenders (Table 8.6).

We consider first the group consisting of blacks only. The predictions for this group, for the 1978 data, are given in Table 8.4. Of the 11 groups

---

[5] If the treatment group were randomly chosen, then there would be no need for a model to test the effect of the treatment, of course.

[6] Recall that PRIORS is the number of previous incarcerations *in addition to* the sample incarceration.

[7] That is, the case in which the model estimated from the 1978 analysis sample is used to make predictions for the listed groups in the 1978 validation sample.

TABLE 8.3. Summary of subsample predictions, logit lognormal model.

	1978			1980			Using 1978 model to predict for 1980	
Subsample	N	χ^2	$\lvert F-\hat{F}\rvert$	N	χ^2	$\lvert F-\hat{F}\rvert$	χ^2	$\lvert F-\hat{F}\rvert$
WHITE = 0	1470	43.0	.017	2106	67.0	.021	74.1	.032
WORKREL = 1	1432	47.4	.027	1846	64.4	.033	75.7	.044
AGE < 252	583	58.3	.066	1008	46.8	.056	115.3	.109
AGE ⩾ 480	387	33.2	.016	566	58.8	.079	63.1	.068
ALCHY = 1	603	34.4	.032	1551	57.8	.042	67.4	.048
JUNKY = 1	838	48.6	.062	845	44.4	.030	58.4	.061
FELON = 1	989	78.2	.052	1778	40.4	.014	153.4	.095
MALE = 0	175	51.1	.023	242	26.0	.047	35.1	.078
PROPTY = 1	792	61.7	.035	1895	68.0	.030	124.3	.077
TSERVD > 12	1508	64.0	.031	2057	111.3	.058	168.3	.083
PRIORS ≠ 0	1310	76.1	.057	1823	92.4	.057	130.6	.076

considered, this is the one for which we predict more accurately. The predictions are generally not as accurate as those for the whole validation sample, however. (Compare the summary statistics in Tables 3.2 and 8.3.) For 1978, we moderately overpredict early recidivism, as can be seen clearly in Table 8.4. For 1980, we underpredict recidivism throughout, and the differences are noticeable if not large. When we use the 1978 model to make predictions for 1980, we again underpredict recidivism throughout; the magnitude of this underprediction is roughly similar to that reported earlier for the entire validation sample.

It is worth emphasizing the result that models estimated for the entire release cohort predict adequately for blacks, and this is consistent with our previous findings (Schmidt & Witte, 1978). Apparently, our models capture the effect of race on recidivism adequately. This implies that it is not necessary to estimate separate models for black releasees in order to obtain accurate predictions for groups consisting entirely or predominantly of blacks.

We next consider the group consisting of individuals who participated in the North Carolina prisoner work release program during their sample sentence. The predictions for this group, for the 1978 data, are given in Table 8.5. These predictions are better than those for most of the other 10 groups considered but not nearly as good as those for the best of them (such as the group of blacks only, just described). For both 1978 and 1980, we underpredict recidivism noticeably (and often significantly), except that we predict reasonably accurately in the tail of the 1978 distribution. When we use the 1978 model to make predictions for 1980, we underpredict recidivism throughout, and the degree of underprediction is again similar to that for the entire validation sample.

The variable WORKREL, which defines this group, was tried as an explanatory variable in our models of Chapters 6 and 7, but it consistently

TABLE 8.4. Predicted versus actual recidivism rates for 1978 validation sample, WHITE = 0 (1,470 individuals), using logit lognormal model.

N	Predicted cdf	cdf	t	Predicted density	Density	t	Predicted hazard	Hazard	t	χ^2	df
0	.000	.000	−.66	.000	.000	−.66	.000	.000	−.66	—	—
1	.005	.007	.94	.005	.007	1.14	.005	.007	1.14	0.9	1
2	.015	.012	−.75	.010	.005	−1.61	.010	.005	−1.60	3.5	2
3	.027	.021	−1.37	.012	.009	−1.19	.012	.009	−1.19	4.9	3
4	.041	.031	−1.80	.014	.010	−1.15	.014	.010	−1.16	6.2	4
5	.055	.039	−2.71	.014	.007	−2.20	.015	.008	−2.23	11.2	5
6	.069	.052	−2.56	.014	.014	−.27	.015	.014	−.33	11.3	6
7	.084	.070	−1.88	.014	.018	1.10	.015	.019	1.03	12.4	7
8	.098	.087	−1.36	.014	.017	.99	.015	.018	.96	13.3	8
9	.111	.099	−1.45	.014	.012	−.44	.015	.013	−.45	13.5	9
10	.124	.114	−1.16	.013	.015	.62	.015	.017	.61	13.8	10
11	.137	.130	−.78	.013	.016	1.04	.014	.018	1.03	14.9	11
12	.149	.144	−.59	.012	.014	.52	.014	.016	.55	15.2	12
13	.161	.159	−.15	.012	.016	1.43	.013	.018	1.50	17.5	13
14	.172	.165	−.66	.011	.006	−1.84	.013	.007	−1.77	20.6	14
15	.182	.173	−.90	.011	.008	−.94	.013	.010	−.88	21.4	15
16	.193	.188	−.49	.010	.014	1.55	.012	.017	1.62	24.0	16
17	.202	.197	−.50	.010	.010	−.11	.012	.012	−.02	24.0	17
18	.212	.205	−.61	.009	.008	−.49	.011	.010	−.40	24.2	18
19	.221	.214	−.68	.009	.008	−.34	.011	.010	−.26	24.2	19
20	.229	.221	−.78	.009	.007	−.47	.011	.010	−.39	24.4	20
21	.238	.231	−.65	.008	.010	.54	.010	.012	.63	24.8	21
22	.246	.241	−.44	.008	.010	.99	.010	.013	1.09	26.0	22
23	.253	.247	−.57	.008	.006	−.65	.010	.008	−.56	26.3	23
24	.261	.255	−.49	.007	.008	.39	.009	.011	.49	26.5	24
25	.268	.265	−.26	.007	.010	1.16	.009	.013	1.27	28.1	25
26	.274	.272	−.19	.007	.007	.35	.009	.010	.46	28.4	26
27	.281	.278	−.28	.006	.005	−.49	.009	.007	−.38	28.5	27
28	.287	.282	−.47	.006	.004	−1.05	.008	.006	−.95	29.4	28
29	.293	.288	−.39	.006	.007	.40	.008	.009	.51	29.7	29
30	.299	.293	−.54	.006	.004	−.86	.008	.006	−.77	30.3	30
31	.304	.296	−.72	.006	.003	−1.11	.008	.005	−1.05	31.4	31
32	.315	.299	−.88	.005	.003	−1.03	.007	.005	−.97	32.3	32

33	.310	.306	−.74	.005	.007	.87	.007	.010	.95	33.2	33
34	.320	.312	−.64	.005	.006	.62	.007	.009	.70	33.7	34
35	.325	.317	−.64	.005	.005	−.03	.007	.007	.06	33.7	35
36	.329	.322	−.63	.005	.005	.07	.007	.007	.15	33.7	36
37	.334	.325	−.72	.004	.003	−.62	.006	.005	−.54	34.0	37
38	.338	.329	−.74	.004	.004	−.15	.006	.006	−.07	34.0	38
39	.342	.335	−.64	.004	.005	.74	.006	.008	.84	34.7	39
40	.346	.338	−.69	.004	.003	−.39	.006	.005	−.32	34.8	40
41	.350	.343	−.62	.004	.005	.52	.006	.007	.60	35.2	41
42	.354	.346	−.70	.004	.003	−.67	.006	.004	−.60	35.5	42
43	.358	.349	−.73	.004	.003	−.17	.005	.005	−.10	35.6	43
44	.361	.351	−.85	.004	.002	−.98	.005	.003	−.93	36.4	44
45	.365	.355	−.80	.003	.004	.41	.005	.006	.48	—	—
46	.368	.360	−.68	.003	.005	.94	.005	.007	1.02	37.5	45
47	.371	.362	−.78	.003	.002	−.81	.005	.003	−.76	—	—
48	.374	.366	−.70	.003	.004	.64	.005	.006	.71	37.5	46
49	.378	.369	−.67	.003	.003	.24	.005	.005	.31	—	—
50	.381	.373	−.63	.003	.003	.31	.005	.005	.38	37.8	47
51	.383	.375	−.70	.003	.002	−.60	.004	.003	−.55	—	—
52	.386	.378	−.65	.003	.003	.44	.004	.005	.50	37.8	48
53	.389	.381	−.65	.003	.003	.01	.004	.004	.06	—	—
54	.392	.383	−.70	.003	.002	−.45	.004	.003	−.41	37.8	49
55	.394	.385	−.74	.003	.002	−.40	.004	.003	−.36	—	—
56	.397	.388	−.67	.002	.003	.70	.004	.006	.74	37.9	50
57	.399	.391	−.64	.002	.003	.23	.004	.004	.27	—	—
58	.401	.394	−.61	.002	.003	.29	.004	.004	.33	38.1	51
59	.404	.395	−.74	.002	.001	−1.29	.004	.001	−1.27	—	—
60	.406	.396	−.81	.002	.001	−.71	.004	.002	−.69	40.0	52
61	.408	.398	−.82	.002	.002	−.11	.004	.003	−.09	—	—
62	.410	.399	−.88	.002	.001	−.63	.003	.002	−.62	40.2	53
63	.412	.402	−.83	.002	.003	.56	.003	.005	.58	—	—
64	.414	.404	−.83	.002	.002	.03	.003	.003	.05	40.4	54
65	.416	.407	−.71	.002	.003	1.25	.003	.006	1.28	—	—
66	.418	.410	−.64	.002	.003	.71	.003	.005	.74	42.5	55
67	.420	.412	−.69	.002	.001	−.45	.003	.002	−.43	—	—
68	.422	.413	−.72	.002	.001	−.41	.003	.002	−.40	42.8	56
69	.424	.416	−.64	.002	.003	.87	.003	.005	.88	—	—
70	.425	.417	−.67	.002	.001	−.34	.003	.002	−.33	43.0	57

TABLE 8.5. Predicted versus actual recidivism rates for 1978 validation sample, WORKREL = 1 (1,432 individuals), using logit lognormal model.

N	Predicted cdf	cdf	t	Predicted density	Density	t	Predicted hazard	Hazard	t	χ^2	df
0	.000	.000	−.61	.000	.000	−.61	.000	.000	−.61	—	—
1	.004	.005	.23	.004	.005	.40	.004	.005	.39	0.1	1
2	.013	.010	−1.05	.008	.005	−1.47	.008	.005	−1.46	2.2	2
3	.024	.022	−.35	.011	.013	.63	.011	.013	.62	2.6	3
4	.036	.034	−.48	.012	.011	−.32	.012	.011	−.32	2.7	4
5	.048	.048	−.06	.013	.015	.69	.013	.015	.69	3.2	5
6	.061	.064	.47	.013	.016	1.11	.013	.017	1.14	4.4	6
7	.074	.084	1.44	.013	.020	2.34	.013	.021	2.40	10.2	7
8	.086	.098	1.66	.012	.015	.79	.013	.016	.91	11.0	8
9	.098	.110	1.46	.012	.011	−.29	.013	.012	−.17	11.1	9
10	.110	.125	1.85	.012	.015	1.33	.013	.017	1.48	13.3	10
11	.121	.138	2.02	.011	.013	.76	.012	.015	.92	14.1	11
12	.132	.151	2.16	.011	.013	.68	.012	.015	.88	14.9	12
13	.142	.162	2.19	.010	.011	.33	.012	.013	.53	15.2	13
14	.152	.173	2.28	.010	.011	.50	.011	.013	.72	15.7	14
15	.161	.184	2.40	.009	.011	.67	.011	.014	.93	16.5	15
16	.170	.197	2.72	.009	.013	1.41	.010	.015	1.72	19.5	16
17	.179	.205	2.57	.009	.008	−.40	.010	.010	−.14	19.5	17
18	.187	.212	2.40	.008	.007	−.55	.010	.009	−.29	19.6	18
19	.195	.218	2.20	.008	.006	−.71	.009	.008	−.47	19.8	19
20	.203	.226	2.24	.008	.008	.33	.009	.011	.61	20.2	20
21	.210	.232	2.05	.007	.006	−.77	.009	.007	.52	20.5	21
22	.217	.236	1.76	.007	.004	−1.28	.008	.005	−1.06	21.6	22
23	.224	.240	1.44	.007	.003	−1.50	.008	.005	−1.30	23.3	23
24	.231	.246	1.41	.006	.006	−.08	.008	.008	.15	23.3	24
25	.237	.251	1.28	.006	.005	−.63	.008	.006	−.42	23.5	25
26	.243	.260	1.56	.006	.009	1.53	.007	.012	1.82	26.8	26
27	.248	.266	1.60	.006	.006	.28	.007	.008	.54	27.1	27
28	.254	.272	1.66	.006	.006	.40	.007	.009	.66	27.5	28
29	.259	.279	1.80	.005	.007	.88	.007	.010	1.16	28.9	29
30	.264	.282	1.58	.005	.003	−1.23	.006	.004	−1.04	29.9	30
31	.269	.284	1.32	.005	.002	−1.53	.006	.003	−1.37	31.8	31
32	.274	.288	1.27	.005	.004	−.30	.006	.006	−.10	31.8	32

33	.279	.291	1.05	.005	.002	−1.39	.006	.003	−1.24	33.3	33
34	.283	.295	1.02	.004	.004	−.13	.006	.006	.07	33.4	34
35	.287	.297	.89	.004	.003	−.85	.006	.004	−.69	33.8	35
36	.291	.302	.96	.004	.005	.46	.005	.007	.67	34.3	36
37	.295	.309	1.15	.004	.006	1.39	.005	.009	1.65	37.0	37
38	.299	.312	1.12	.004	.003	−.21	.005	.005	−.02	37.0	38
39	.303	.316	1.10	.004	.003	−.14	.005	.005	.06	—	—
40	.306	.318	.97	.004	.002	−.94	.005	.003	−.79	37.3	39
41	.310	.321	.91	.003	.003	−.44	.005	.004	−.27	—	—
42	.313	.323	.80	.003	.002	−.83	.005	.003	−.68	37.7	40
43	.317	.326	.82	.003	.003	.16	.004	.005	.34	—	—
44	.320	.329	.79	.003	.003	−.24	.004	.004	−.09	37.8	41
45	.323	.332	.76	.003	.003	−.18	.004	.004	−.02	—	—
46	.326	.336	.87	.003	.004	.86	.004	.006	1.05	38.3	42
47	.329	.337	.74	.003	.001	−1.04	.004	.002	−.93	—	—
48	.331	.341	.80	.003	.003	.51	.004	.005	.68	38.3	43
49	.334	.344	.86	.003	.003	.58	.004	.005	.75	—	—
50	.337	.348	.94	.003	.003	.64	.004	.005	.82	39.6	44
51	.339	.348	.72	.003	.000	−1.91	.004	.000	−1.84	—	—
52	.342	.352	.86	.002	.004	1.31	.004	.006	1.49	39.6	45
53	.344	.353	.72	.002	.001	−1.32	.003	.001	−1.23	—	—
54	.346	.353	.58	.002	.001	−1.28	.003	.001	−1.20	42.6	46
55	.349	.354	.45	.002	.001	−1.25	.003	.001	−1.18	—	—
56	.351	.356	.44	.002	.002	−.09	.003	.003	.01	43.3	47
57	.353	.359	.49	.002	.003	.53	.003	.004	.65	—	—
58	.355	.361	.49	.002	.002	.01	.003	.003	.11	43.6	48
59	.357	.362	.44	.002	.001	−.53	.003	.002	−.45	—	—
60	.359	.365	.51	.002	.003	.70	.003	.004	.82	43.6	49
61	.361	.369	.64	.002	.003	1.35	.003	.006	1.49	—	—
62	.363	.372	.72	.002	.003	.80	.003	.004	.93	46.6	50
63	.365	.373	.68	.002	.001	−.38	.003	.002	−.30	—	—
64	.367	.374	.65	.002	.001	−.34	.003	.002	−.26	46.7	51
65	.368	.376	.68	.002	.002	.33	.003	.003	.43	—	—
66	.370	.377	.59	.002	.001	−.91	.003	.001	−.86	46.8	52
67	.372	.380	.69	.002	.003	1.07	.003	.004	1.17	—	—
68	.373	.381	.67	.002	.001	−.20	.002	.002	−.13	47.4	53
69	.375	.383	.66	.002	.001	−.16	.002	.002	−.09	—	—
70	.376	.384	.65	.002	.001	−.13	.002	.002	−.06	47.4	54

failed to have a coefficient that was statistically significant at usual confidence levels. It therefore was not included in the final specification. As a result, it seems unlikely that the significant underprediction of recidivism that we find here is actually due to program effects (which, it should be noted, would then be *negative*, indicating that participation in a work release program worsened post-release behavior). More likely, the problem is that work release participants have different characteristics than nonparticipants, and our model does not adequately capture the effects of these characteristics on time until recidivism. An obvious next step would be to try to identify these characteristics and to enter them into the model in ways that more adequately capture their effects.

The third group that we will discuss in detail is the group of youthful offenders. These are individuals who are less than 21 years old (AGE < 252). Of the 11 groups we consider, this is the one for which we predict most poorly. The predictions for this group, for the 1978 data, are presented in Table 8.6. In all cases, we underpredict recidivism quite considerably. For example, when we use the 1978 model to make predictions for the 1978 validation sample (Table 8.6), the predicted proportion of recidivists after 24 months is .237 whereas the actual proportion is .287. For 1980, the same figures are .298 and .347; when we use the 1978 model to make predictions for 1980, they become .249 and .347. These are very serious underpredictions, and they would tend to make any program for young offenders appear to be ineffective (or actually counterproductive). The variable AGE is an important one in our model, and it appears that we have not adequately captured its effect on time until recidivism by simply entering it linearly into the specification. Whether we require a more flexible form for the effect of age (e.g., quadratic), or interactions with other variables, or even a separate model for youthful offenders, is an open question of some importance.

One pattern that is apparent in our predictions is a tendency to predict better for larger groups. This should be expected, as the model is known to predict well for the entire validation sample.

Our results in making predictions for nonrepresentative subsamples are not very satisfactory. Our model predicted quite well for the entire cohort, with little evidence of significant prediction errors. For the subsamples just considered, however, the model predicts much more poorly, and there are many prediction errors that are statistically significant at usual confidence levels for almost all of the groups. This casts serious doubt on the model's usefulness in program evaluation, but it also suggests a rich agenda for future research.

Individual Predictions

In this section, we use our statistical models to make predictions of recidivism for individuals, rather than just for groups. This is a fairly standard use of such models; for example, the studies in Farrington and Tarling (1985) include predictions of failure on parole, of recidivism, and of absconding from institutions for young offenders. The desire to make predictions for individuals undoubtedly derives from a desire to use such predictions as the basis for differential treatments for individuals. For example, the policy of selective incapacitation, which has been advocated by Greenwood (1982) and others, would involve lengthening the prison terms of those individuals who are predicted to be future failures (recidivists), perhaps combined with more lenient treatment of those individuals who are not predicted to be future failures. The success of such a policy hinges on the ability to predict accurately which individuals will and will not fail and, therefore, which individuals should be selectively incapacitated or selectively deinstitutionalized. Thus the accuracy of our predictions for individuals is of central importance.

Because our data are on the length of time until recidivism,[8] it is natural for us to regard recidivism as the event to be predicted and to ask how well our models predict it. Recidivism is a discrete (yes/no) event, whereas our models yield a *probability*, between zero and one, of this event for each individual. This immediately raises the question of how to summarize the accuracy of the models' predictions.[9] One possibility is to use statistical measures (akin to correlations) of the degree of association between the models' probabilities and the observed binary outcome. Though Kendall's tau has often been suggested for this purpose, a more standard statistical measure would be the biserial correlation coefficient, which is a form of the correlation coefficient used when one variable is continuous and the other is binary. However, we will not pursue such measures here, as they are not of obvious practical use.

A more readily interpreted summary of predictive success, in the present context, is to predict that individuals with probabilities above some chosen level will return to prison (and that individuals with probabilities below that level will not) and to calculate the error rate of these predictions. This seems reasonable because it evaluates the accuracy of the exact procedure that would be followed in a practical application of these models. We need to distinguish two types of errors: "false positives," which are individuals who are predicted to return to prison but do not, and "false negatives," which are individuals who are predicted not to return to prison but do return.

We then encounter the question of how high the probability of recidivism must be before we predict that the individual will be a recidivist (or how low it must be to predict the opposite). One obvious possibility is to predict recidivism for all individuals for whom the model's probability of

---

[8] With recidivism defined as return to prison in North Carolina.

[9] The methods we pursue here are quite standard. See Blumstein et al. (1986), Farrington and Tarling (1985), and Gottfredson and Tonry (1987).

TABLE 8.6. Predicted versus actual recidivism rates for 1978 validation sample, AGE < 252 (583 individuals), using logit lognormal model.

N	Predicted cdf	cdf	t	Predicted density	Density	t	Predicted hazard	Hazard	t	χ^2	df
0	.000	.000	−.40	.000	.000	−.40	.000	.000	−.40	—	—
1	.005	.002	−1.03	.004	.002	−.96	.004	.002	−.96	1.1	1
2	.013	.005	−1.71	.009	.003	−1.36	.009	.003	−1.37	2.9	2
3	.024	.021	−.60	.011	.015	.99	.011	.016	.96	3.9	3
4	.037	.036	−.10	.012	.015	.66	.013	.016	.65	4.3	4
5	.050	.046	−.39	.013	.010	−.57	.013	.011	−.57	4.6	5
6	.063	.065	.23	.013	.019	1.22	.014	.020	1.22	6.1	6
7	.076	.077	.12	.013	.012	−.21	.014	.013	−.18	6.1	7
8	.089	.101	1.07	.013	.024	2.44	.014	.026	2.49	12.3	8
9	.101	.118	1.40	.012	.017	1.05	.013	.019	1.15	13.7	9
10	.113	.134	1.61	.012	.015	.78	.013	.018	.90	14.5	10
11	.124	.151	1.96	.011	.017	1.29	.013	.020	1.43	16.5	11
12	.135	.172	2.57	.011	.021	2.21	.012	.024	2.42	22.4	12
13	.146	.189	2.95	.011	.017	1.55	.012	.021	1.80	25.6	13
14	.156	.192	2.42	.010	.003	−1.62	.011	.004	−1.48	27.8	14
15	.166	.202	2.40	.010	.010	.14	.011	.013	.34	27.9	15
16	.175	.221	2.96	.009	.019	2.41	.011	.024	2.72	—	—
17	.184	.232	3.00	.009	.010	.36	.010	.013	.61	33.5	16
18	.192	.238	2.84	.009	.007	−.44	.010	.009	−.22	—	—
19	.201	.252	3.14	.008	.014	1.49	.010	.018	1.81	34.8	17
20	.208	.262	3.24	.008	.010	.68	.009	.014	.97	—	—
21	.216	.268	3.06	.008	.005	−.66	.009	.007	−.43	34.9	18
22	.223	.274	3.01	.007	.007	−.10	.009	.009	.16	—	—
23	.230	.280	2.88	.007	.005	−.51	.008	.007	−.29	34.9	19
24	.237	.285	2.76	.007	.005	−.44	.008	.007	−.22	—	—
25	.243	.297	3.06	.006	.012	1.71	.008	.017	2.07	36.6	20
26	.249	.302	2.98	.006	.005	−.30	.008	.007	−.06	—	—
27	.255	.314	3.30	.006	.012	1.93	.007	.017	2.33	39.2	21
28	.261	.321	3.35	.006	.007	.39	.007	.010	.69	—	—
29	.266	.323	3.31	.005	.005	−.10	.007	.008	.16	39.5	22
30	.271	.334	3.48	.005	.009	1.11	.007	.013	1.46	—	—
31	.276	.338	3.37	.005	.003	−.55	.007	.005	−.33	40.2	23
32	.281	.341	3.27	.005	.003	−.50	.006	.005	−.28	—	—

33	.286	.350	3.47	.005	.009	1.37	.006	.013	1.73	41.2	24
34	.291	.357	3.58	.005	.007	.84	.006	.011	1.17	—	—
35	.295	.360	3.52	.004	.003	−.34	.006	.005	−.11	41.8	25
36	.299	.365	3.55	.004	.005	.34	.006	.008	.63	—	—
37	.303	.369	3.51	.004	.003	−.24	.005	.005	−.01	42.0	26
38	.307	.369	3.29	.004	.000	−1.52	.005	.000	−1.40	—	—
39	.311	.374	3.35	.004	.005	.52	.005	.008	.81	42.2	27
40	.315	.376	3.23	.004	.002	−.78	.005	.003	−.61	—	—
41	.318	.381	3.31	.004	.005	.64	.005	.008	.93	42.2	28
42	.322	.383	3.21	.003	.002	−.71	.005	.003	−.54	—	—
43	.325	.386	3.20	.003	.003	.04	.005	.006	.27	42.3	29
44	.328	.388	3.12	.003	.002	−.65	.004	.003	−.48	—	—
45	.331	.391	3.13	.003	.003	.13	.004	.006	.36	42.3	30
46	.334	.395	3.14	.003	.003	.17	.004	.006	.41	—	—
47	.337	.400	3.25	.003	.005	.98	.004	.008	1.28	43.7	31
48	.340	.405	3.36	.003	.005	1.04	.004	.009	1.35	—	—
49	.343	.407	3.30	.003	.002	−.49	.004	.003	−.31	44.2	32
50	.346	.408	3.25	.003	.002	−.45	.004	.003	−.28	—	—
51	.348	.410	3.20	.003	.002	−.42	.004	.003	−.25	44.4	33
52	.351	.410	3.06	.003	.000	−1.22	.004	.000	−1.12	—	—
53	.353	.410	2.93	.002	.000	−1.20	.004	.000	−1.11	46.9	34
54	.356	.412	2.89	.002	.002	−.34	.003	.003	−.17	—	—
55	.358	.417	3.03	.002	.005	1.41	.003	.009	1.72	48.0	35
56	.360	.420	3.09	.002	.003	.59	.003	.006	.84	—	—
57	.363	.424	3.15	.002	.003	.63	.003	.006	.88	49.5	36
58	.365	.424	3.03	.002	.000	−1.12	.003	.000	−1.03	—	—
59	.367	.425	3.01	.002	.002	−.20	.003	.003	−.02	50.1	37
60	.369	.425	2.91	.002	.000	−1.09	.003	.000	−1.00	—	—
61	.371	.427	2.89	.002	.002	−.14	.003	.003	.03	50.6	38
62	.373	.427	2.79	.002	.000	−1.06	.003	.000	−.98	—	—
63	.375	.431	2.87	.002	.003	.87	.003	.006	1.12	50.6	39
64	.376	.432	2.86	.002	.002	−.06	.003	.003	.11	—	—
65	.378	.439	3.12	.002	.007	2.91	.003	.012	3.35	56.5	40
66	.380	.439	3.02	.002	.000	−1.01	.003	.000	−.92	—	—
67	.382	.439	2.94	.002	.000	−.99	.003	.000	−.91	58.2	41
68	.383	.443	3.03	.002	.003	1.06	.002	.006	1.33	—	—
69	.385	.443	2.94	.002	.000	−.97	.002	.000	−.89	58.3	42
70	.386	.443	2.86	.002	.000	−.96	.002	.000	−.88	—	—

recidivism is at least .5 and to predict nonrecidivism for all individuals for whom the probability is less than .5. This is not necessarily a good idea when the sample proportion of recidivists is not close to .5. For example, if recidivism is a fairly rare event, even a good model may imply a probability of recidivism that is less than .5 for almost every individual; conversely, if recidivism is a very common event, the model may imply a probability of recidivism greater than .5 for almost every individual. An alternative rule (e.g., Wilbanks, 1985) is that the proportion of individuals predicted to fail should be equal to the proportion of the group that we expect to fail. For example, in our 1978 estimation sample, the failure rate is .366; by this rule, then, we would predict recidivism for the 36.6% of the validation sample who have the highest probabilities of recidivism, regardless of the absolute magnitudes of these probabilites. Basing our predictions on the proportional hazards model, we would predict recidivism for 1,127 individuals (36.6% of the 3,078 individuals in the 1978 validation sample). Of this number, 595 actually returned to prison and 532 did not. We would also predict that 1,951 individuals would not to return to prison; 540 of this number returned to prison and 1411 did not. We therefore have a false positive rate of 532/1127 = .472 and a false negative rate of 540/1951 = .277.

The predictive accuracy of our models compares quite favorably with the accuracy of the models recently surveyed by Farrington (1987). He reports that Greenwood (1982) had a false positive rate of 56% and a false negative rate of 46% for his estimation sample (Greenwood had no validation sample). Our false positive rate is approximately 10% lower and our false negative rate approximately 20% lower than Greenwood's. This is particularly impressive because our predictions are for a validation sample rather than an estimation sample. Janus (1985), whose predictions resulted in an even poorer record, had a 62% false positive rate and a 64% false negative rate. Blumstein, Farrington, and Moitra (1985) found a false negative rate of 35%, which is lower than that of either Greenwood or Janus, although almost 10% higher than our own; their false positive rate is higher than either Greenwood's or ours. It is clear that we are able to predict more accurately than the studies surveyed by Farrington. However, our false positive rate is still much too high to allow one to feel comfortable with using our models to pick individuals for selective incapacitation.

On the other hand, in some cases, neither of the rules discussed above may be appropriate. For example, in considering a policy of selective incapacitation, a false positive rate of 47% is clearly unacceptable, but we might be satisfied if we could predict recidivism with considerable assurance for even a very limited proportion of the sample. For example, if 10% of the release cohort had probabilities of recidivism that were nearly equal to one, we might feel justified in selectively incapacitating these individuals, regardless of what the model might predict for other individuals in the sample. We will therefore report the accuracy of our predictions for many different values of the proportion of individuals whom we predict to fail, and the reader can choose which results are interesting.

We will begin with the individual predictions of recidivism for the 1978 validation sample that are implied by the proportional hazards model, when it is estimated using data from the 1978 estimation sample. These results are given in Table 8.7. Recall that the proportional hazards model yields a "score" for each individual; in the notation of Chapter 6, the score for individual i is of the form $\mathbf{X}_i\boldsymbol{\beta}$. This score can be converted into a probability of recidivism, but we will note simply that the probability is higher when the score is higher (and, of course, the converse is true). We therefore rank individuals by their scores and calculate the proportions of individuals who fail in various percentiles of the score distribution. As noted earlier, this seems to be the information that is most likely to be useful in potential applications, such as contemplating a policy of selective incapacitation.

Looking at Table 8.7, it is clear that the model has at least some predictive power, as the individuals in the upper tail of the score distribution do indeed fail more often than the individuals in the lower tail. For example, for the 308 individuals who represent the highest-scoring 10% of the sample, the failure rate is 66.6%; the 308 individuals who represent the lowest-scoring 10% of the population, on the other hand, have a failure rate of only 13.3%. Similarly, the highest-scoring 50% of the sample has a failure rate of 48.1%, compared with 25.6% for the lowest-scoring 50% of the sample, and so forth.

In considering a policy of selective incapacitation, it is important that there is some group of individuals whom we can predict to fail with near certainty. Using this model, any such group would have to be very small. For example, the highest-scoring 0.5% of the sample has a recidivism rate of 86.7%, but it is a group of only 15 individuals. The recidivism rate falls to 80.6% if we double the size of the group to include the 31 individuals in the upper 1% of the score distribution, and it falls to 70.1% if we include the 154 individuals in the upper 5% of the score distribution. The probabilities of a false positive error implied by these recidivism rates seem rather high; a public official who is considering selective incapacitation for the "worst" 1% of a potential release cohort probably would not like to think that 20% of those "worst" individuals would in fact not return to prison after a 4-year follow-up.

We are much more successful in predicting individuals who will *not* fail. For example, in the group of 31 individuals who represent the lowest-scoring 1% of the sample, the failure rate is only 3.2% (only one such individual fails). Even if we enlarge the group considerably to include the 308 individuals who are the lowest-scoring 10% of the sample, the failure rate is only 13.3%; this false negative rate is much lower than the corresponding false positive rate (33.4%) for the corresponding upper 10% of scores. It is clear that predictions of the type made here need to be used

TABLE 8.7. Individual predictions for 1978 validation sample using proportional hazards model.

Upper percentile	Number	% Recidivists	Average score	Lower percentile	Number	% Recidivists	Average score
0%	0	—	—	100%	3078	36.9	−.2843
.5%	15	86.7	1.8110	99.5%	3063	36.6	−.2946
1%	31	80.6	1.6040	99%	3047	36.4	−.3035
5%	154	70.1	1.0180	95%	2924	35.1	−.3529
10%	308	66.6	.7528	90%	2770	33.6	−.3996
20%	616	58.8	.5036	80%	2462	31.4	−.4815
30%	923	55.6	.3556	70%	2155	28.9	−.5584
40%	1231	51.9	.2517	60%	1847	26.9	−.6416
50%	1539	48.1	.1646	50%	1539	25.6	−.7333
60%	1847	46.1	.0811	40%	1231	23.0	−.8326
70%	2155	43.8	.0036	30%	923	20.8	−.9565
80%	2462	41.8	−.0720	20%	616	17.0	−1.1330
90%	2770	39.5	−.1586	10%	308	13.3	−1.4150
95%	2924	38.5	−.2116	5%	154	6.5	−1.6660
99%	3047	37.2	−.2651	1%	31	3.2	−2.1770
99.5%	3063	37.0	−.2740	.5%	15	6.7	−2.3390
100%	3078	36.9	−.2843	0%	0	—	—

with considerable caution. However, even at the current state of development, the individual predictions of recidivism generated by our models may be useful to prison classification committees considering placement in lower security facilities, home visits, or placement on work or study release. They may also be of interest to the parole board when it is deciding whether to release an inmate before the expiration of his or her term. However, it is certainly true that predictions of future behavior should be only one of a number of types of information taken into account when decisions affecting inmates are made.

Table 8.8 is very similar to Table 8.7. It simply covers the predictions for 1980 rather than 1978. These are similar enough to not require a separate discussion.

Table 8.9 contains the same information as Table 8.7, except that the variables WHITE and MALE are not included in calculating the individual scores. In any practical application of predictions from models such as these, it is not clear exactly which variables would be considered appropriate for inclusion. For example, one presumably cannot refuse to parole an individual because he is black, even though being black leads to a higher score from our models. We do not attempt to answer here the question of which individual characteristics might legitimately be used to determine differential treatment of individuals. Others have considered this issue at length. For example, see Morris and Miller (1985), Blumstein et al. (1986), and Tonry (1987). Opinions differ. However, many people would agree that it is inappropriate to allow either race or sex to affect the treatment that individuals receive.

To accommodate these very legitimate concerns, we delete WHITE and MALE to see how much predictive accuracy is lost by deleting from the scoring function a few variables that were significant predictors of recidivism. Interestingly, there is little if any such loss of predictive ability (compare Tables 8.5 and 8.7). This is perhaps surprising, as WHITE was a very significant predictor of time until recidivism in all of our models containing individual characteristics.

The results given so far are all from the proportional hazards model of Chapter 6. Table 8.10 gives the same results but from the logit lognormal model of Chapter 7. These results are so similar to those just discussed that they do not need separate discussion. In other words, the choice of model does not seem to make much difference in the quality of the individual predictions. This is perhaps to be expected, as the choice of model did not make much difference in the estimated effects of individual characteristics on time until recidivism. It is a potentially important finding, however, because it suggests that researchers who are interested primarily in individual predictions may be able to use fairly standard models and readily available statistical packages (for example, SAS and BMDP contain a program for the proportional hazards model) without a substantial loss of predictive ability.

TABLE 8.8. Individual predictions for 1980 validation sample using proportional hazards model.

Upper percentile	Number	% Recidivists	Average score	Lower percentile	Number	% Recidivists	Average score
0%	0	—	—	100%	4304	36.8	−.3029
.5%	22	81.8	1.6340	99.5%	4282	36.5	−.3128
1%	43	81.4	1.4410	99%	4261	36.3	−.3205
5%	215	69.8	.9322	95%	4089	35.0	−.3678
10%	430	61.2	.7396	90%	3874	34.0	−.4186
20%	861	56.4	.5429	80%	3443	31.8	−.5144
30%	1291	53.2	.4166	70%	3013	29.7	−.6111
40%	1722	49.4	.3119	60%	2582	28.4	−.7129
50%	2152	46.6	.2207	50%	2152	27.0	−.8265
60%	2582	45.0	.1321	40%	1722	24.4	−.9551
70%	3013	42.7	.0434	30%	1291	22.8	−1.1110
80%	3443	40.6	−.0507	20%	961	21.4	−1.3110
90%	3874	38.7	−.1560	10%	430	19.1	−1.6260
95%	4089	37.9	−.2189	5%	215	14.9	−1.9010
99%	4261	37.1	−.2815	1%	43	2.3	−2.4220
99.5%	4282	36.9	−.2913	.5%	22	0.0	−2.5660
100%	4304	36.8	−.3029	0%	0	—	—

TABLE 8.9. Individual predictions for 1978 validation sample using proportional hazards model, without WHITE or MALE.

Upper percentile	Number	% Recidivists	Average score	Lower percentile	Number	% Recidivists	Average score
0%	0	—	—	100%	3078	36.9	−.7168
5%	15	73.3	1.3150	99.5%	3063	36.7	−.7268
1%	31	83.9	1.0550	99%	3047	36.4	−.7349
5%	154	71.4	.5042	95%	2924	35.1	−.7811
10%	308	61.4	.2459	90%	2770	34.2	−.8239
20%	616	57.0	−.0058	80%	2462	31.8	−.8947
30%	923	52.5	−.1480	70%	2155	30.2	−.9605
40%	1231	50.1	−.2548	60%	1847	28.0	−1.0250
50%	1539	49.0	−.3389	50%	1539	24.8	−1.0950
60%	1847	45.9	−.4077	40%	1231	23.3	−1.1810
70%	2155	43.7	−.4694	30%	923	20.9	−1.2950
80%	2462	41.3	−.5336	20%	616	19.3	−1.4490
90%	2770	39.4	−.6081	10%	308	14.0	−1.6950
95%	2924	38.2	−.6534	5%	154	11.0	−1.9210
99%	3047	37.2	−.6994	1%	31	0.0	−2.4260
99.5%	3063	37.1	−.7074	5%	15	0.0	−2.6440
100%	3078	36.9	−.7168	0%	0	—	—

TABLE 8.10. Individual predictions for 1978 validation sample using logit lognormal model.

Upper percentile	Number	% Recidivists	Average score	Lower percentile	Number	% Recidivists	Average score
0%	0	—	—	100%	3078	36.9	−.0980
.5%	15	80.0	4.7340	99.5%	3063	36.7	−.1217
1%	31	83.9	4.0750	99%	3047	36.4	−.1405
5%	154	70.1	2.5670	95%	2924	35.1	−.2384
10%	308	67.5	1.9200	90%	2770	33.5	−.3224
20%	616	59.9	1.3350	80%	2462	31.1	−.4565
30%	923	55.9	1.0180	70%	2155	28.7	−.5760
40%	1231	53.5	.7987	60%	1847	25.8	−.6956
50%	1539	50.3	.6291	50%	1539	23.5	−.8252
60%	1847	47.0	.4833	40%	1231	21.6	−.9703
70%	2155	44.2	.3474	30%	923	19.8	−1.1380
80%	2462	42.2	.2203	20%	616	15.7	−1.3700
90%	2770	39.5	.0860	10%	308	13.0	−1.7530
95%	2924	38.4	.0058	5%	154	8.4	−2.0690
99%	3047	37.2	−.0714	1%	31	6.5	−2.7100
99.5%	3063	37.0	−.0838	.5%	15	6.7	−3.0010
100%	3078	36.9	−.0980	0%	0	—	—

The results of this section can be summarized as follows. Our models imply a probability of recidivism for each individual (and for each length of time since release). The models have predictive power in the sense that individuals with high implied probabilities of recidivism do indeed return to prison more often than individuals with low probabilities. The real question is whether the degree of predictive power is high enough to make the models useful for decision-makers. As noted previously, we believe the models are good enough to allow predictions based on them to be used *as one piece of information* among many to select inmates for more favourable treatment. For example, the 10% of our sample with the lowest scores had a recidivism rate of only 13%, whereas the highest-scoring 10% of our sample had a recidivism rate of almost 70%. We have succeeded in identifying a relatively low risk group of individuals. However, we have been much less successful in identifying a group that is sufficiently sure to return to prison that we might be justified in selectively incapacitating them. Of course, this clearly depends on how large a false positive rate one is willing to tolerate. Our models' false positive rates are rather high: about 20% even for the 1% of the sample with the highest predicted probabilities of recidivism, and over 30% for the top 10% of the sample. We personally find these rates to be too high to use our models for selecting individuals for harsher treatment than they would receive otherwise.

This is not to say that formal models like ours are necessarily useless in this context. Perhaps our model could be improved with further work; we have given earlier some suggestions for such improvements. Also, our definition of recidivism (return to prison in North Carolina) is obviously restrictive, and models fit to data that support a less restrictive definition of recidivism (e.g., rearrest) may be more successful. (Certainly, they should suffer from less of a problem with false positives, but presumably they would suffer from more of a problem with false negatives.) Finally, we stress that we are making no comment on the likely justification of a policy of selective incapacitation; we are only expressing pessimism about the usefulness of our models for establishing such a justification. A policy of selective incapacitation would be far easier to market if there were some "objective" scientific evidence of one's power to identify a particularly crime-prone group of individuals. We have been able to identify such a group but only with a level of error that we feel is unacceptable.

Conclusions

In this chapter, we have considered predictions of recidivism for individuals, as well as for groups of individuals that differ systematically in their characteristics from the sample on which the estimation of the model was based. These types of predictions require models that contain individual characteristics as explanatory variables.

Our predictions of recidivism for groups of individuals were of mixed quality. We first used four models fit to data from the 1978 estimation sample to make predictions for the 1980 validation sample. These predictions were reasonably good; our best 1978 model predicted recidivism in the 1980 validation sample almost as well as our best 1980 model. Our interpretation of this result is that most of the difference in recidivism rates across the 2 years is explained by differences in observable characteristics of the releasees. However, when we used our best 1978 model to make predictions for clearly nonrandom subsamples of the 1978 validation sample (such as blacks, alcoholics, felons, and so forth), the results were much less favorable. We predicted rather poorly for many of these groups. The apparent explanation is that our model does not adequately capture the effects of individual characteristics on time until recidivism. We have entered such characteristics into our models linearly (for example, in the logit lognormal model, the logit portion of the model is linear in the explanatory variables), and the logical next step would be to try some more flexible functional forms. Because many of the coefficients in our models are highly statistically significant, there is reason to hope that the data will indeed support a more flexible parameterization.

Our predictions of recidivism for individuals are reasonable in the sense that individuals with high predicted probabilities of recidivism do return to prison more often than individuals with low predicted probabilities of recidivism. However, the degree of predictive power is not as high as we might hope. In particular, though we can predict quite accurately which individuals will not return to prison, we have trouble predicting with any certainty which individuals will do so. Our failure to predict more precisely is not a question of the adequacy of the model in the sense discussed above. Rather, it is simply a reflection of the fact that the proportion of the variability of time until recidivism that is explained by the model is low. As reported in Chapter 7, the effective R^2 (proportion of variability explained) of our models is only about .1. Individual predictions of recidivism that are accurate enough to provide an objective, scientific justification for a policy of selective incapacitation will have to come from models with a higher degree of explanatory power than ours.

9
Summary and Conclusions

Summary

The purpose of this study was to investigate the usefulness of various statistical survival time models for prediction of the length of time that a prison releasee will remain free after release from incarceration. In particular, we were interested in the following three issues. First, we wished to compare the results from parametric statistical models with those from nonparametric models. Second, we wished to examine the importance of including individual characteristics as explanatory variables in such models. Third, we wished to examine the usefulness of so-called split models, in which not every individual would eventually return to prison.

We used data for two cohorts of individuals released from prison in North Carolina: our 1978 data set, which consists of all individuals released from North Carolina prisons between July 1, 1977 and June 30, 1978, and our 1980 data set, which consists of all individuals released from North Carolina prisons between July 1, 1979 and June 30, 1980. Recidivism was determined by a search of North Carolina Department of Correction records in April 1984, so that the follow-up times ranged from 46 to 81 months. A complete description of the data is given in Chapter 2.

The nature of the data required recidivism to be defined as return to prison in North Carolina, which is obviously a less than ideal definition for most purposes. (It is, however, the definition most likely to be of interest to the North Carolina Department of Correction.) It is also clearly the case that, by limiting our analyses to North Carolina data, we have no basis for judging the extent to which our conclusions can be generalized to other jurisdictions. However, the data have some very good features. First, they contain detailed information on a large number of individuals. There are approximately 9,500 individuals in each year's data set, and we used information on 15 individual characteristics as explanatory variables. (A list of these explanatory variables is given in the section Definitions of Variables in Chapter 2.) Furthermore, this information has been computerized and subjected to a variety of checks for internal consistency, and it is as accurate as any data we can reasonably hope for. Second, data are available on more than one cohort, with consistent definitions of variables, so we can check the extent of behavioral change over time. Third, the length of the follow-up is much longer than is usually the case in criminal justice research.

The dependent variable that we have analyzed is time until recidivism, defined more precisely as the length of time from an individual's release from prison until his or her return to prison in North Carolina. From a statistical point of view, this is a "survival time" (or "failure time") analysis, and our statistical methodology follows directly from that statistical literature. We give a survey of this methodology in Chapter 3.

It is now widely recognized that the length of time until recidivism is a much more useful variable than the simpler yes/no measure of recidivism for some fixed time after release, and there are two reasons for this. First, the timing of recidivism contains useful information; from a statistical point of view, it is inefficient to ignore this. Second, once we have estimated the distribution of time until recidivism, we can make predictions of the rate of recidivism for any period of time after release, not just for the particular follow-up period found in the data used to estimate the model.

To investigate the accuracy of our models and their predictions, we follow the common practice of dividing our basic samples of data randomly into two subsamples: an "estimation sample," which we use to estimate the models, and a "validation sample," for which we make predictions.[1] Since the division of the data into estimation and validation samples is random, significant differences between the two samples should occur only by chance.[2] In general, we would expect the models that best fit the estimation sample to best predict for the validation sample. (Indeed, this is basically what we found.) However, it is commonly the case that models provide a better fit to the data on which they are estimated than they do for other similar data, such as our validation samples. This phenomenon is called "shrinkage," a good discussion of which can be found in Copas (1985). The more flexibly parameterized a model is, the larger its shrinkage tends to be. (Making a model more flexible by adding another parameter

[1] The records of some individuals in our basic samples lacked information on one or more variables used in our analyses. These observations were discarded, and the observations with complete information were randomly split into an estimation sample and a validation sample for each cohort. Thus, for each cohort, there is actually a third sample, consisting of individuals with missing data, which is not used at all. This is described in more detail in Chapter 2.

[2] Unfortunately, there is a statistically significant difference in the average time until recidivism between the 1980 estimation and validation samples, which is due simply to bad luck in the random division of the 1980 complete data sample. This makes the job of predicting for the 1980 validation sample more difficult than it otherwise would be. However, it does provide an unusually stringent test for our model.

will always improve the fit to the estimation sample, but this will not necessarily improve the predictions for the validation sample.) The number of parameters in our models ranges widely, from one to 19. The use of a validation sample is therefore potentially important to avoid an overparameterized model.

We first considered, in Chapter 4, models of time until recidivism that did not use individual characteristics as explanatory variables. Until quite recently, the survival time models used in criminal justice research have not used explanatory variables. For example, see Maltz (1984) for a thorough treatment of such models. We felt that it was important to consider a wide variety of models without explanatory variables, so we could get a good idea of how accurately they could predict recidivism in our data. This provides an obvious benchmark to measure the accuracy of the predictions from our (later) models that included explanatory variables.

The first model that we considered was a nonparametric "model," which simply predicted, for each of the two validation samples, that the proportion of recidivists in each month would be the same as in the corresponding estimation sample. Given that the estimation and validation samples were formed by a random division of the original sample, these predictions should not contain systematic errors (bias). For the 1978 data, they did not. However, the recidivism rates found in the 1980 estimation sample underpredicted the corresponding recidivism rates in the 1980 validation sample. This difference in recidivism between the 1980 estimation and validation samples is just the result of an unluckly random split of the data into the two samples.

However, the real defect of the nonparametric predictions was that they were too noisy, in that they varied too much from month to month. (Figure 4.1 provides an illustration of this fact.) There was therefore an obvious possibility of improving predictions by "smoothing" the recidivism rate in the estimation sample before making predictions. This is precisely what is accomplished by assuming a parametric statistical model, as any probability distribution we assume would have a relatively smooth density or hazard function. (For example, see Figure 4.2.) However, a parametric model can yield predictions that are biased (systematically wrong) if the model is not adequate, and the losses due to this bias have to be weighed against the gains from removing the excess noise of nonparametric predictions. This makes it very important to investigate the adequacy of the models that one assumes.

We next considered parametric statistical models that did not use explanatory variables. Specifically, we considered models based on the exponential, lognormal, log-logistic, Weibull, and LaGuerre distributions. All of these except the LaGuerre are distributions commonly considered in the failure time literature. The exponential model has been most extensively used in criminal justice applications, although the lognormal and Weibull models also have been used. Unfortunately, as we report in

Chapter 4, none of these distributions fit our data adequately, and none yielded predictions that were better than our nonparametric predictions. See Table 3.2 for a summary. The apparent reason is that our data have features not commonly found in typical failure time applications (such as failure times of machines or survival times of medical patients). Specifically, in our data the hazard rate is not monotonic; it first rises, and then falls. Furthermore, once it begins to fall, it falls quite quickly because very few individuals who have not returned to prison within two or three years do so later. Our simple models of time until recidivism could not adequately capture this type of variation in recidivism rates. They all tended to overpredict recidivism for the period immediately after release, underpredict recidivism for the next year or so, and then overpredict recidivism again for periods long after release.

We next considered split models in the sense of Maltz and McCleary (1977). In a split model, it is assumed that not all individuals will eventually return to crime, and the probability of eventual recidivism is an additional parameter to be estimated. The distribution that is assumed for time until recidivism is understood to be relevant only for the fraction of the sample that will eventually fail; that is, the distribution is *conditional* on eventual recidivism. The methodological virtue of such split models is that they imply a rapidly falling hazard rate (at least in the tail of the distribution), thus matching an important feature of our data. Their substantive value is that they allow one to estimate the "ultimate" probability or rate of recidivism or, equivalently, the termination rate. This is an important theoretical concept which can also be of practical use in, for example, making projections of future prison populations.

As we report in Chapter 5, we tried the same five distributions (exponential, lognormal, log-logistic, Weibull, and LaGuerre) for our split models as we had previously considered for the simple models of Chapter 4. The best model we found was the split lognormal model, which apparently has not been used previously in criminal justice research. The split lognormal model's fit to the 1978 estimation sample and its predictions for the 1978 validation sample were entirely adequate. (See Figure 5.1 and compare it with Figure 4.2.) It also fit the 1980 estimation sample adequately. Its predictions for the 1980 validation sample were less satisfactory, but they were probably as good as could be expected, given the difference in recidivism rates between the 1980 estimation and validation samples.

Combining information from our study with the results of the few studies with long follow-up periods that have been conducted, it appears that the ultimate probability of recidivism for prison releasees may be approximately 50%. It is interesting that the ultimate rate of recivivism may be less than 20% higher than the 3-year rate commonly reported. The rate of recidivism (hazard rate) declines markedly over time, and our follow-up is long enough to reveal this clearly.

The first model we considered that used individual characteristics as explanatory variables was the proportional hazards model, described in Chapter 6. It allows one to estimate the effects of such variables on time until recidivism without having to assume a particular form for the distribution of survival times. This model has recently gained some popularity in criminal justice research. Because the distribution of the survival times is modeled in a nonparametric way, the proportional hazards model is not very useful for predicting the timing of return to prison. However, as we note in Chapter 8, the proportional hazards model is about as good as any other model we consider at predicting *which* individuals will eventually return to prison.

Our main interest in the proportional hazards model was to see which individual characteristics had significant effects on time until recidivism, without making a specific distributional assumption. This was of interest in its own right, and it was a preliminary step in the specification of our parametric models with explanatory variables. However, we also wished to assess the predictive accuracy of the proportional hazards model so that it could be used as a benchmark to judge our parametric models.

Our results for the 1978 and 1980 cohorts were quite similar. They indicate that the type of individual most likely to recidivate is a young, black male who is a drug addict and/or alcoholic, who has a large number of previous incarcerations, and whose previous incarceration was lengthy and for a crime against property. These results are quite similar to the results of previous studies of recidivism. A possible exception is the effect of race. However, the effect of race on recidivism appears to be quite unstable; see Chapter 6 for a discussion.

We next turned to parametric statistical models with explanatory variables. Our results for these models are reported in Chapter 7. We considered models based on the exponential, lognormal, and LaGuerre distributions. These were allowed to be split distributions, with the explanatory variables affecting both the probability of eventual recidivism and the mean time until recidivism for the eventual recidivists. We believe that the models of Chapter 7 represent a significant methodological innovation of wide potential usefulness. They bring together two different strains of the criminological literature using survival analysis. The first such strain, developed mainly by Maltz and his colleagues (e.g., Maltz & McCleary, 1977; Maltz, 1984), developed split models but did not use explanatory variables. The second strain, developed by Schmidt and Witte (1977, 1984), and others, used explanatory variables but did not consider split models. By combining these two approaches, we can attempt to separate the influences of explanatory variables on the probability of (eventual) recidivism from their influences on the timing of recidivism for the eventual recidivists.

The estimated effects of individual characteristics on recidivism for the parametric models were very similar to those described above for the proportional hazards model, regardless of which distribution was assumed. It was easier to find significance for the effects of individual characteristics on the probability of eventual recidivism than for their effects on mean time until recidivism. However, we had some trouble distinguishing these two effects of explanatory variables, in the sense that this distinction was not robust to the choice of distribution.[3]

In spite of these somewhat disappointing results, we believe that it is worthwhile to continue the development of models (like our models of Chapter 7) that distinguish the effects of explanatory variables on the probability of recidivism from their effects on the timing of recidivism. This distinction is very important if we are to understand the factors leading an individual to "drop out" of crime, as well as the factors leading to various rates of crime commission for those who continue in a life of crime. It would be quite interesting to estimate such models using data for general population groups such as birth cohorts (e.g., the 1945 and 1958 Philadelphia birth cohorts). Because of the longer time span over which individuals may be observed in birth-cohort data, we can presumably observe individuals ceasing to participate in criminal activities with greater assurance than in our shorter data sets; we can also observe the timing of recidivism in much more detail. Therefore, we might hope to better distinguish factors that affect eventual recidivism from factors that affect its timing. Further, analysis of such data sets will allow us to discern the factors affecting the decision ever to participate in criminal activity.

Not surprisingly, the choice of distribution is important for the quality of the predictions for our validation samples. The lognormal models were far superior to those based on the exponential distribution. Our best model was the logit lognormal model, in which individual characteristics affect the probability of eventual recidivism according to a logit model, with time until recidivism (for the eventual recidivists) following a lognormal distribution with constant mean and variance. This model predicted the recidivism of the 1978 and 1980 validation samples as well as, but no better than, the split lognormal model that did not contain explanatory variables. (Compare Figures 5.1 and 7.1.) Thus the use of individual characteristics as explanatory variables did not result in improved predictions for random samples of releasees. This was unexpected. The variance of time until recidivism should be reduced by conditioning on relevant explanatory variables, and thus better predictions were anticipated when such variables were included in the model. However, our models fit the data rather loosely; they explained only about 10% of the variation in time until recidivism. Such a level of explanatory power is common in studies of recidivism. However, we believe that further work with models of the type

[3] For example, for 1980, the property crime variable (PROPTY) affected the probability of recidivism, but not its timing, in the lognormal model. The opposite was true in the exponential model.

developed here could lead to substantial improvement in the fit of survival models to recidivism data. Clearly, a noticeable improvement in predictive ability will require better-fitting models.

We also considered the use of our models to make predictions for individuals and nonrandom samples of releasees. These results are reported in Chapter 8. The first question addressed is whether models fit to the 1978 data can predict accurately the recidivism rate in the 1980 data. Models that do not contain explanatory variables cannot do so. Because the recidivism rate is higher in the 1980 data than in the 1978 data, models that did not contain explanatory variables and that were fit to the 1978 data always underpredicted the recidivism rate in the 1980 data. On the other hand, our best model containing explanatory variables (the logit lognormal model) predicted the recidivism experience in the 1980 validation sample about as well when fit to the 1978 estimation sample as when fit to the 1980 estimation sample. (See Table 3.2.) In that sense, differences across the cohorts in the values of observable individual characteristics accounted for virtually all of the observed difference in recidivism rates across the cohorts. This is encouraging for the practical usefulness of such models, as they presumably would be of limited interest if they could be used only to make predictions for the cohort on which they were estimated.

We next considered the accuracy of predictions for nonrandom samples of releasees, such as youthful offenders, property offenders, or participants in North Carolina's prisoner work release program. These results were rather discouraging. For most groups that we considered, the predicted rates of recidivism differed substantially and significantly from the actual recidivism rates. This finding casts serious doubt on our models' usefulness in program evaluation using the "predicted versus actual" method suggested in our earlier work (Schmidt & Witte, 1980, 1984). The apparent problem is that our models do not capture adequately the effects of the explanatory variables on time until recidivism. Perhaps this could be solved by a richer specification of these effects. For example, instead of having all variables enter linearly into the logit portion of the logit lognormal model, we might consider interactions, quadratic terms, and so forth. In our previous work, we were able to improve the predictive accuracy of our models substantially by estimating separate models for different sex, age, and race groups, and perhaps we could do so in our present models as well. However, all we can really say at present is that, without further work to improve the fit of our models, our ability to make accurate predictions for nonrandom samples of releasees is rather limited.

Finally, we used our models that contained explanatory variables to make predictions of recidivism for individuals. The quality of these predictions did not seem to depend much on which model was used. For example, the results for the proportional hazards model were very similar to those for the logit lognormal model. (Compare Tables 8.9 and 8.10.) These predictions were reasonable, in the sense that individuals with large implied probabilities of recidivism did indeed return to prison more often than individuals with low probabilities. The predictive power of our models was good by the standards of a number of recent studies (e.g., Blumstein et al., 1985; Greenwood, 1982) and exceeded Farrington's (1987) criterion for a well-designed prediction study. Still, our false positive rate of 47% is worrisome. Such a level of false positives clearly casts serious doubt on the use of statistical methods of prediction, at their current state of development, to implement a policy of selective incapacitation. Our false negative rate of 28% is more acceptable, suggesting that statistical prediction at this point may be more useful for selecting individuals for favorable treatment (e.g., probation or parole) than selecting them for treatment that is particularly harsh.

Conclusions

The purpose of the research reported here was to explore the usefulness of various statistical survival time models. We were particularly interested in exploring three issues: (1) the relative merits of parametric and nonparametric methods, (2) the usefulness of explicitly incorporating explanatory variables into the models, and (3) the effect of including a splitting parameter. We evaluated the usefulness of the various models that we estimated by assessing the quality of their predictions. Our predictions, though reasonably good by the standards of previous work, were not entirely satisfactory. Clearly, much work remains to be done. We hope that our research has given others an indication of which lines of work are likely to be productive.

We believe that we have demonstrated convincingly the usefulness of parametric statistical models. Purely nonparametric models generate predictions with too much statistical noise to be of much use. Random variations over time in the recidivism rate cry out for some sort of smoothing prior to prediction, and this is what a statistical model can achieve. We were able to find models (such as our split lognormal model) that fit the samples on which they were estimated quite well and that generated better predictions for random samples of releasees than was possible nonparametrically. On the other hand, we tried many different models before we found such an adequate model; we considered five different distributions and still had to use a split model to fit the data well. Though our best models were quite good, our worst models were woefully inadequate and produced predictions that were systematically and seriously in error. It is certainly not advisable to pick a particular model (e.g., Weibull, split exponential, or proportional hazards) just because it can be found in a statistics book or because software is available to fit it. Indeed, we found most models with readily available software to be inadequate for our data, and it took a great deal of effort for us to find any model that we regarded as adequate. The lesson is clear: although parametric models are clearly useful, it is up to the investigator to investigate and justify the adequacy of his or her model.

Our attempts to demonstrate the usefulness of individual characteristics as explanatory variables in such models were less successful. Our successes were as follows. We were able to obtain statistically significant and believable results for the effects of individual characteristics on time until recidivism. These results were robust to different distributional assumptions, which is certainly comforting. We were able to predict quite adequately for random samples of releasees. Furthermore, we could do so even when we used the model estimated on data from one cohort (1978) to make predictions for a different release cohort (1980) with a higher recidivism rate.

On the other hand, we failed in some other respects. We were unable to improve our predictions for random samples of releasees (from the same release cohort as the estimation sample) by using individual characteristics as explanatory variables. We were unable to predict accurately for most nonrandom samples of releasees. Our predictions were good for some such groups but awful for others. Finally, our predictions for individuals were reasonable. However, they suffered from a high false positive rate. We were not able to accurately identify a group of career criminals who might be selectively incapacitated. Our false negative rate was lower, and in that sense, we were able to identify a group that usefully might be considered for fewer restrictions on their freedom. The predictions of our model would be more useful for implementing a policy of selective deinstitutionalization than of selective incapacitation.

Incorporation of a splitting parameter into our models greatly improved our ability to predict the timing of recidivism. It appears that it is important to incorporate this parameter to adequately reflect the rapid decrease in the hazard rate after the first few months. Split models imply that certain individuals would *never* recidivate, and this insight is of considerable theoretical and practical interest. Theoretically, it can help us sort out the effects of explanatory variables on the decision to participate in crime, as opposed to their effects on the rate of participation. Practically, it can help us to analyze and predict both the frequency and the duration of criminal careers.

It is an open question whether our failures could be reversed with further work. Each of them is related to the failure of our models to capture adequately the effects of individual characteristics on time until recidivism. Each of our models embodies a distributional assumption, plus some assumptions about the functional form of the effects of the explanatory variables on the dependent variable. For example, in our logit lognormal model, the probability of eventual recidivism is assumed to follow a logit model; individual characteristics are assumed to enter the logit model linearly; and the distribution of time until recidivism (conditional on eventual recidivism) is assumed to be lognormal. In this project, we devoted a huge amount of effort to finding the "best" distributional assumptions to make, by trying many different distributions and checking the adequacy of the resulting predictions over time. We devoted much less effort to investigating the proper ways to enter individual characteristics into our models; they were always simply entered linearly somewhere or other in the model. The fact that our models predicted adequately for random samples of releasees, but not for nonrandom samples such as youthful offenders or property offenders, strongly suggests that we need a more adequate representation of the ways in which characteristics like age and nature of previous offense affect outcomes. Of course, it is not clear without further analysis of the data precisely what sorts of complications (group specific models, quadratics, interactions, transformations of variables, etc.) are likely to be useful, but the ease with which we found significance for a rather large set of variables suggests that the data may indeed support such complications. If so, there is hope that some version of our models would turn out to predict accurately for nonrandom samples of releasees, as well as for the entire validation sample.

With respect to our failure to improve our predictions for random samples of releasees by using explanatory variables, or to predict as accurately as we would like for individuals, different but related considerations apply. Here the problem is not that the predictions are systematically wrong, but that they are just too imprecise. This is true simply because the proportion of the variation in time until recidivism that is explained by the model is low, with the equivalent of R^2 being only about 10%. What we need is basically just a better-fitting model. Of course, it is clear that expanding the model to capture more adequately the effects of individual characteristics on the dependent variable should make the model fit better, thus improving the quality of predictions for individuals and random samples of releasees (as well as for nonrandom samples of releasees). What is not clear is how successful such an attempt is likely to be. Even if we doubled the R^2 from .1 to .2, there would still be considerable unexplained variation (noise) in the model, and it may be presumptuous to expect the resulting predictions to improve markedly. Nevertheless, the importance of being able to make better predictions is so great that this is a task worth undertaking.

In order to facilitate further research, we have made our data available in machine-readable form from the Interuniversity Consortium on Political and Social Research (ICPSR) at the University of Michigan.

References

Adler, I., & Kandel, D.B. (1983). Risk periods for drug involvement in adolescence in France and Israel: Application of survival analysis to cross-sectional data. *Social Forces*, *62*, 375–397.

Amemiya, T., & Boskin, M. (1974). Regression analysis when the dependent variable is truncated lognormal, with an application to the duration of welfare dependency. *International Economic Review*, *15*, 485–496.

Anscombe, F.J. (1961). Estimating a mixed-exponential response law. *Journal of the American Statistical Association*, *56*, 493–502.

Barton, R.R., & Turnbull, B.W. (1981). A failure rate regression model for the study of recidivism. In J.A. Fox (Ed.), *Models in quantitative criminology*. New York: Academic Press.

Berk, R.A., & Rauma, D. (1983). Capitalizing on random assignment to treatments: A regression–discontinuity evaluation of a crime-control program. *Journal of the American Statistical Association*, *78*, 21–27.

Black, T., & Spinks, P. (1985). Predicting outcomes of mentally disordered and dangerous offenders. In D.P. Farrington and R. Tarling (Eds.), *Prediction in criminology*. Albany: State University of New York Press.

Bloom, H.S. (1979). Evaluating human service and correctional programs by modeling the timing of recidivism. *Sociological Methods and Research*, *8*, 179–208.

Blumstein, A., Cohen, J., Martin, S., & Tonry, M. (1983). *Research on sentencing: The search for reform*. Washington, DC: National Academy Press.

Blumstein, A., Cohen, J., Roth, J.A., & Visher, C.A. (1986). *Criminal careers and "career criminals."* Washington, DC: National Academy Press.

Blumstein, A., Farrington, D., & Moitra, S. (1985). Delinquency careers: Innocents, desisters and persisters. *Crime and Justice: An Annual Review of Research*, *7*, 187–220.

Brannas, K., & Eklof, J.A. (1985). *Criminal policy and recidivism—An empirical study on Swedish data*. Working paper, Department of Statistics, University of Umea.

Burgess, E.W. (1928). Factors determining success or failure on parole. In A.A. Bruce, E.W. Burgess, & A.J. Harno, *The workings of the indeterminate sentence law and the parole system in Illinois*. Springfield: Illinois State Board of Parole.

Carr-Hill, G.A., & Carr-Hill, R.A. (1972). Reconviction as a process. *British*

Journal of Criminology, *12*, 35–43.
Carr-Hill, R.A., & Stern, N.H. (1979). *Crime, the police and criminal statistics*. London: Academic Press.
Chaiken, J.M., & Rolph, J.E. (1981). Methods for estimating crime rates of individuals (Report No. R-2730-NIJ). Santa Monica, CA: Rand Corporation to the National Institute of Justice.
Collins, J.S. (1986). The relationship of problem drinking to individual offending sequences. In A. Blumstein et al. (Eds.), *Criminal careers and "career criminals"* (Vol. 2). Washington, DC: National Academy Press.
Copas, J.B. (1985). Prediction equations, statistical analysis, and shrinkage. In D.P. Farrington and R. Tarling (Eds.), *Prediction in criminology*. Albany: State University of New York Press.
Cox, D.R. (1972). Regression models and life tables. *Journal of the Royal Statistical Society*, *Series B*, *34*, 187–220.
Cox, D.R. (1975). Partial likelihood. *Biometrika*, *62*, 276–296.
Cox, D.R., & Oates, D. (1984). *Analysis of survival data*. London: Chapman and Hall.
Farrington, D.P. (1979). Longitudinal research on crime and delinquency. *Crime and Justice: An Annual Review of Research*, *1*, 289–348.
Farrington, D.P. (1985). Predicting self-reported and official delinquency. In D.P. Farrington and R. Tarling (Eds.), *Prediction in criminology*. Albany: State University of New York Press.
Farrington, D.P. (1987). Predicting individual crime rates. *Crime and Justice: An Annual Review of Research*, *9*, pp. 53–102.
Farrington, D.P., & Tarling, R. (1985). Criminological prediction: The way forward. In D.P. Farrington and R. Tarling (Eds.), *Prediction in criminology*. Albany: State University of New York Press.
Farrington, D.P., & Tarling, R. (1985). *Prediction in criminology*. Albany: State University of New York Press.
Farrington, D.P., Ohlin, L.E., & Wilson, J.Q. (1986). *Understanding and controlling crime: Toward a new research strategy*. New York: Springer-Verlag.
Flinn, C. (1986). Dynamic models of criminal careers. In A. Blumstein et al. (Eds.), *Criminal careers and "career criminals"* (Vol. 2). Washington, DC: National Academy Press.
Ghali, M.A. (1982). The choice of crime: An empirical analysis of juveniles' criminal choice. *Journal of Criminal Justice*, *10*, 433–442.
Glueck, S., & Glueck, E.T. (1950). *Unraveling juvenile delinquency*. Cambridge, MA: Harvard University Press.
Goldfeld, S.M., & Quandt, R.E. (1981). Econometric modelling with non-normal disturbances. *Journal of Econometrics*, *17*, 41–156.
Gottfredson, S.D. (1987). Prediction: An overview of selected methodological issues. *Crime and Justice: An Annual Review of Research*, *9*, pp. 21–52.
Gottfredson, S.D., & Gottfredson, D.M. (1985). Screening for risk among parolees: Policy, practice and method. In D.P. Farrington and R. Tarling (Eds.), *Prediction in Criminology*. Albany: State University of New York Press.
Gottfredson, S.D., & Gottfredson, D.M. (1986). Accuracy of prediction models. In A. Blumstein et al. (Eds.), *Criminal careers and "career criminals"* (Vol. 2). Washington, DC: National Academy Press.
Gottfredson, D.M., & Tonry, M. (1987). *Crime and Justice: An Annual Review of*

Research, *9*.
Greenberg, D.F. (1978). Recidivism as radioactive decay. *Journal of Research in Crime and Delinquency*, *15*, 124–125.
Greenwood, P. (1982). *Selective incapacitation*. Santa Monica, CA: Rand Corporation.
Harris, C.M., Kaylan, A.R., & Maltz, M.D. (1981). Refinements in the statistics of recidivism measurement. In J.A. Fox (Ed.), *Models in quantitative criminology*. New York: Academic Press.
Harris, C.M., & Moitra, S. (1978). Improved statistical techniques for the measurement of recidivism. *Journal of Research in Crime and Delinquency*, *15*, 194–213.
Hoffman, P.B., & Stone-Meierhoefer, B. (1979). Post release arrest experiences of federal prisoners: A six-year follow-up. *Journal of Criminal Justice*, *7*, 193–216.
Janus, M.C. (1985). Selective incapacitation: Have we tried it? Does it work? *Journal of Criminal Justice*, *13*, 117–129.
Kalbfleisch, J.D., & Prentice, R.L. (1980). *The statistical analysis of failure time data*. New York: Wiley.
Kiefer, N.M. (1985). Specification diagnostics based on LaGuerre alternatives for econometric models of duration. *Journal of Econometrics*, *28*, 135–154.
Kitchener, H., Schmidt, A.K., & Glaser, D. (1977). How persistent is post-prison success? *Federal Protection, 41*, 9–15.
Lawless, J.F. (1982). *Statistical models and methods for lifetime data*. New York: Wiley.
Lloyd, M.R., & Joe, G.W. (1979). Recidivism comparison across groups: Methods of estimation and tests of significance for recidivism rates and asymptotes. *Evaluation Quarterly*, *3*, 105–111.
Lutkepohl, H. (1980). Approximation of arbitrary distributed lag structures by a modified polynomial lag: An extension. *Journal of the American Statistical Association*, *75*, 428–430.
Maltz, M.D. (1978). Comments on "Stability of parameter estimates in the split population exponential distribution." *Evaluation Quarterly*, *2*, 650–654.
Maltz, M.D. (1984). *Recidivism*. Orlando, FL: Academic Press.
Maltz, M.D., & McCleary, R. (1977). The mathematics of behavioral change: Recidivism and construct validity. *Evaluation Quarterly*, *1*, 421–438.
Maltz, M.D., McCleary, R., & Pollock, S.M. (1979). Recidivism and likelihood functions: A reply to Stollmack. *Evaluation Quarterly*, *3*, 124–131.
Martin, S.E., Sechrest, L.B., & Redner, R. (1981). *The rehabilitation criminal offenders: New directions for research*. Washington, DC: National Academy of Sciences.
McCord, J. (1978). A thirty year follow-up of treatment effects. *American Psychologist*, 284–289.
Menard, S., & Covey, H. (1983). Community alternatives and rearrest in Colorado. *Criminal Justice and Behavior*, *10*, 93–108.
Miley, A.D. (1978). Stability of parameter estimates in the split population exponential distribution. *Evaluation Quarterly*, *2*, 646–649.
Monahan, J. (1981). *Predicting violent behavior: An assessment of clinical techniques*. Beverly Hills, CA: Sage Publications.
Morris, N., & Miller, M. (1985). On "dangerousness" in the judicial process. *Crime and Justice: An Annual Review of Research*, *7*, 1–50.

Petersilia, J., & Turner, S. (1987). Guideline-based justice: Implications for racial minorities. *Crime and Justice: An Annual Review of Research*, *9*, pp. 151–182.

Peto, R. (1972). Contribution to the discussion of paper by D.R. Cox. *Journal of the Royal Statistical Society, Series B*, *34*, 472–475.

Prentice, R.L. (1973). Exponential models with censoring and explanatory variables. *Biometrika*, *60*, 279–288.

Rhodes, W., & Matsuba, S. (1985). *A survival model with dependent competing events and right-hand censoring: Probation and parole as an illustration*. Working paper, Inslaw, Inc., Washington, DC.

Schmidt, P., & Mann, W.R. (1977). A note on the approximation of arbitrary distributed lag structures by a modified Almon lag. *Journal of the American Statistical Association*, *72*, 442–443.

Schmidt, P., & Witte, A.D. (1976). *Determinants of criminal recidivism*. Report to the North Carolina Department of Correction.

Schmidt, P., & Witte, A.D. (1978). *Determinants of criminal recidivism: Further investigations*. Report to the North Carolina Department of Correction.

Schmidt, P., & Witte, A.D. (1979). Models of criminal recidivism and an illustration of their use in evaluating correctional programs. In L. Sechrest, S. White, & E. Brown (Eds.), *The rehabilitation of criminal offenders: Problems and prospects*. Washington, DC: National Academy of Sciences.

Schmidt, P., & Witte, A.D. (1980). Evaluating correctional programs: Models of criminal recidivism and an illustration of their use. *Evaluation Review*, *4*, 585–600.

Schmidt, P., & Witte, A.D. (1984). *An economic analysis of crime and justice: Theory, methods, and applications*. Orlando, FL: Academic Press.

Sechrest, L., White, S., & Brown, E. (1979). *The rehabilitation of criminal offenders: Problems and prospects*. Washington, DC: National Academy of Sciences.

Service, P. (1972). *The recidivism of persons released from facilities of the North Carolina Department of Correction during January–July 1968*. Raleigh, NC: North Carolina Department of Correction.

Sherman, L.W., & Berk, R.A. (1984). The specific deterrent effects of arrest for domestic assault. *American Sociological Review*, *49*, 261–271.

Stein, W.E., & Lloyd, M.R. (1981). The Maltz–McCleary model of recidivism: A reexamination. *Evaluation Review*, *5*, 132–144.

Stollmack, S., & Harris, C.M. (1974). Failure rate analysis applied to recidivism data. *Operations Research*, *23*, 1192–1205.

Stone, M.H. (1962). A generalized Weierstrass approximation theorem. In R.C. Buck (Ed.), *Studies in modern analysis* (Vol. 1). Englewood Cliffs, NJ: Prentice Hall.

Tauchen, G., Tauchen, H., & Witte, A.D. (1986). *The dynamics of domestic violence: A reanalysis of the Minneapolis experiment*. Working paper, Department of Economics, Wellesley College.

Tonry, M. (1987). Prediction and classification: Legal and ethical issues. *Crime and Justice: An Annual Review of Research*, *9*, pp. 367–414.

Tracy, P.E., Wolfgang, M.E., & Figlio, R.M. (1985). *Delinquency in two birth cohorts*. Washington, DC: U.S. Department of Justice.

Weis, J.G. (1986). Issues in the measurement of criminal careers. In A. Blumstein et al. (Eds.), *Criminal careers and "career criminals"* (Vol. 2). Washington, DC:

National Academy Press.
Wilbanks, W.L. (1985). Predicting failure on parole. In D.P. Farrington and R. Tarling (Eds.), *Prediction in criminology*. Albany: State University of New York Press.
Wilkins, L.T. (1985). The politics of prediction. In D.P. Farrington and R. Tarling (Eds.), *Prediction in criminology*. Albany: State University of New York Press.
Wilson, J.Q., & Herrnstein, R.J., (1985). *Crime and human nature*. New York: Simon and Schuster.
Wish, E.D., & Johnson, B.D. (1986). The impact of substance abuse on criminal careers. In A. Blumstein et al. (Eds.), *Criminal careers and "career criminals"* (Vol. 2). Washington, DC: National Academy Press.
Witte, A.D. (1975). *Work release in North Carolina: An evaluation of its post-release effects*. Chapel Hill, NC: Institute for Research in Social Science.
Witte, A.D. (1980). Estimating the economic model of crime with individual data. *Quarterly Journal of Economics*, *94*, 57–87.
Witte, A.D., & Schmidt, P. (1977). An analysis of recidivism, using the truncated lognormal distribution. *Applied Statistics*, *26*, 302–311.
Witte, A.D., Woodbury, D.F., Smith, S.H., Barreto, H., & Beaton, R. (1982). *The effect of a less coercive internal prison environment and gradual reintegration on post-release prison performance: An evaluation of Morris' model of imprisonment as implemented at the Federal Correctional Institution at Butner, N.C.* (Contract No. J100c–047). Washington, DC: Federal Bureau of Prisons.

Author Index

Subject Index

MIX
Papier aus verantwortungsvollen Quellen
Paper from responsible sources
FSC® C105338

If you have any concerns about our products,
you can contact us on
ProductSafety@springernature.com

In case Publisher is established outside the EU,
the EU authorized representative is:
Springer Nature Customer Service Center GmbH
Europaplatz 3, 69115 Heidelberg, Germany

Printed by Libri Plureos GmbH
in Hamburg, Germany